CONTENTS

INTRODUCTION

What is a Wood Pellet Grill & Smoker?

A pellet grill runs a bit differently than your traditional gas, charcoal or propane grills. Our Silverbac wood pellet grill and Grilla smoker grill use pellets made of compacted wood for fuel which are fed to a fire pot by an auger. An rod starts the flame and a fan pushes the smoke upwards to spread heat and smoke. A digital control allows you to control the temperature. These components require electricity, so you'll need an outlet to run your smoker grill. Learn more about pellet grills.

Why would I Buy a Wood Pellet Grill &Smoker?

Wood pellet smoker grills take the ease of grilling with gas but give your food that awesome flavor of real wood. Think Crock pot of the grilling world. Slow cooking, set it and forget it controls means you can visit with guests and family and not have to worry about standing over a hot grill turning your food every few minutes. The temperature controls will keep you within degrees of your set temperature, so just dial up your desired temperature and go grab a cold beverage!

How to Use a Wood Pellet Smoker to Smoke Meat

Using a pellet grill is easy with a little practice. There are a few simple tips any aspiring pit boss should be mindful of:

Keep your smoker clean.

A big appeal of cooking with wood pellets is that they burn clean. Don't cancel out this asset by letting charred waste build up in your grill. After each cooking session, take some time to clean up by scraping grill grates and removing unused pellets from the hopper. Use your own temperature probe. Many of today's pellet smokers come with a meat probe, but this can be one of the lowest-quality components of the whole device. Invest in a high-quality digital thermometer, and be precise about cooking at your desired temperature.

Experiment with hardwoods.

In addition to developing a custom dry rub or wet brine, you can work toward creating your own custom blend of hardwoods. Perhaps you're a purist and would never blend one type of wood with another. Or, perhaps you'll find success using pellets from a base wood like hickory, alder, or mesquite, then adding pellets made from fruit wood such as apple or cherry. As a general rule, beef smokes well with all woods except for apple. Chicken tastes great smoked with anything other than oak and maple. Fish is particularly tasty when smoked with alder, oak, or mesquite. Veggies can taste great when smoked over hickory, pecan, and maple wood. And pork works with nearly everything other than mesquite and oak.

Give yourself plenty of cooking space.

While you don't want your smoker to overwhelm your patio, make sure you find one with a large enough cooking area that you can prepare your meats with precision. A good pellet grill can range from just over 200 square inches to well over 800 square inches, so think about your ambitions and choose accordingly. At the end of the day, it's better to have a grill that's a little too large rather than a little too small, but some situations (such as tailgating) are going to mandate a smaller cooker.

Use a sear box.

Pellet smokers do not get nearly as hot as standard charcoal or gas BBQ grills. If you're looking for a single device that can handle both pellet smoking and traditional searing, consider getting a pellet grill that comes with an add-on sear box—essentially a mini grill that can produce temperatures far higher than the smoker itself.

Advantages of The Wood Pellet Grills:

Supremely convenient

Once you have filled up the hopper with pellets, and set the temperature, all you need to do is kick back, relax and wait for your dinner.

Fuel efficient, cheap to run

Pellet grills have a convection fan, meaning they run very efficiently. This means you can expect to spend less on pellets than you would on charcoal.

Easy to maintain

Unlike charcoal grills, pellet grills don't make much of a mess. Aside from the cooking surfaces themselves, you may need to clean out the fire pot occasionally, but that is it.

Versatile

Pellet grills allow you to smoke, roast, bake, barbecue and grill (although the sear won't be as good as you can expect from a charcoal grill) all within the one unit.

Quick

You can expect your pellet grill to be up to temperature and ready to cook within 15 minutes.

FAQs on Your Wood Pellet Grill & Smoker

Are pellet smokers as good as wood smokers?

So, unlike the offset smoker, pellet smokers don't require so much babysitting to low-and-slow a brisket to perfection. But, they do require access to power and, hard-core enthusiasts will say that the results from a pellet smoker are slights less smoky and a bit more moist than what you get off a traditional smoker.

Does my grill require electricity to operate?

The short answer is yes. Your grill must be plugged into an electrical source in order to operate. Electricity powers the controller, the auger, and the induction fan, which are all necessary in operating the grill.

How much electricity does the grill use?

This varies depending on how long the grill has been on. For the first five minutes, the grill will use about 150 watts of electricity, during which time it is lighting the pellets. After the pellets are lit, or after about five minutes, electricity use will drop to less than 100 watts. The searing station uses 1000 watts when it is in use.

What size generator is required to operate my grill?

A 2000-watt generator is recommended for searing station-equipped models, while a 1000-watt generator is sufficient for those without a searing station.

VEGETABLE & VEGETARIAN RECIPES

1. Roasted Hasselback Potatoes

Servings: 6   Cooking Time: 30 Minutes
Ingredients:
- 6 large russet potatoes
- 1-pound bacon
- ½ cup butter
- Salt to taste
- 1 cup cheddar cheese
- 3 whole scallions, chopped

Directions:
Fire the   Grill to 350F. Use desired   wood pellets when cooking. Close the lid and preheat for 15 minutes. Place two wooden spoons on either side of the potato and slice the potato into thin strips without completely cutting through the potato.   Chop the bacon into small pieces and place in between the cracks or slices of the potatoes.   Place potatoes in a cast iron skillet. Top the potatoes with butter, salt, and cheddar cheese.   Place the skillet on the grill grate and cook for 30 minutes. Make sure to baste the potatoes with melted cheese 10 minutes before the cooking time ends.

Nutrition Info: Calories per serving: 662;
Protein: 16.1g; Carbs: 71.5g; Fat: 38g Sugar: 2.3g

2. Grilled Asparagus With Wild Mushrooms

Servings: 4   Cooking Time: 10 Minutes
Ingredients:
- 2 bunches fresh asparagus, trimmed
- 4 cups wild mushrooms, sliced
- 1 large shallots, sliced into rings
- Extra virgin oil as needed
- 2 tablespoons butter, melted

Directions:
Fire the   Grill to 500F. Use desired   wood pellets when cooking. Close the lid and preheat for 15 minutes. Place the asparagus, mushrooms, and shallots on a baking tray. Drizzle with oil and butter and season with salt and pepper to taste.   Place on a baking tray and cook for 10 minutes. Make sure to give the asparagus a good stir halfway through the cooking time for even browning.

Nutrition Info: Calories per serving: 218;
Protein: 15.2g; Carbs: 26.6 g; Fat: 10g Sugar: 12.9g

3. Smoked Healthy Cabbage

Servings: 5   Cooking Time: 2 Hours
Ingredients:
- 1 head cabbage, cored
- 4 tablespoons butter
- 2 tablespoons rendered bacon fat
- 1 chicken bouillon cube
- 1 teaspoon fresh ground black pepper
- 1 garlic clove, minced

Directions:
Preheat your smoker to 240 degrees Fahrenheit using your preferred wood   Fill the hole of your cored cabbage with butter, bouillon cube, bacon fat, pepper and garlic   Wrap the cabbage in foil about two-thirds of the way up   Make sure to leave the top open Transfer to your smoker rack and smoke for 2 hours Unwrap and enjoy!

Nutrition Info: Calories: 231 Fats: 10g Carbs: 26g
Fiber: 1g

4. Shiitake Smoked Mushrooms

Servings: 4-6   Cooking Time: 45 Minutes
Ingredients:
- 4 Cup Shiitake Mushrooms
- 1 tbsp canola oil
- 1 tsp onion powder
- 1 tsp granulated garlic
- 1 tsp salt
- 1 tsp pepper

Directions:
Combine all the ingredients together   Apply the mix over the mushrooms generously.   Preheat the smoker at 180°F. Add wood chips and half a bowl of water in the side tray.   Place it in the smoker and smoke for 45 minutes.   Serve warm and enjoy.

Nutrition Info: Calories: 301 Cal Fat: 9 g
Carbohydrates: 47.8 g   Protein: 7.1 g Fiber: 4.8 g

5. Roasted Spicy Tomatoes

Servings: 4   Cooking Time: 1 Hour And 30 Minutes
Ingredients:
- 2 lb. large tomatoes, sliced in half
- Olive oil
- 2 tablespoons garlic, chopped
- 3 tablespoons parsley, chopped
- Salt and pepper to taste
- Hot pepper sauce

Directions:
Set the temperature to 400 degrees F.   Preheat it for 15 minutes while the lid is closed.   Add tomatoes to a baking pan.   Drizzle with oil and sprinkle with garlic, parsley, salt and pepper.   Roast for 1 hour and 30 minutes.   Drizzle with hot pepper sauce and serve.
Tips: You can also puree the roasted tomatoes and use as sauce for pasta or as dip for chips.

6. Mexican Street Corn With Chipotle Butter

Servings: 4   Cooking Time: 12 To 14 Minutes
Ingredients:

- 4 ears corn
- ½ cup sour cream
- ½ cup mayonnaise
- ¼ cup chopped fresh cilantro, plus more for garnish
- Chipotle Butter, for topping
- 1 cup grated Parmesan cheese

Directions:

Supply your smoker with wood pellets and follow the manufacturer's specific start-up procedure. Preheat, with the lid closed, to 450°F. Shuck the corn, removing the silks and cutting off the cores. Tear four squares of aluminum foil large enough to completely cover an ear of corn. In a medium bowl, combine the sour cream, mayonnaise, and cilantro. Slather the mixture all over the ears of corn. Wrap each ear of corn in a piece of foil, sealing tightly. Place on the grill, close the lid, and smoke for 12 to 14 minutes. Remove the corn from the foil and place in a shallow baking dish. Top with chipotle butter, the Parmesan cheese, and more chopped cilantro. Serve immediately.

7. Wood Pellet Smoked Asparagus

Servings: 4   Cooking Time: 1 Hour
Ingredients:
- 1 bunch fresh asparagus, ends cut
- 2 tbsp olive oil
- Salt and pepper to taste

Directions:

Fire up your wood pellet smoker to 230°F   Place the asparagus in a mixing bowl and drizzle with olive oil. Season with salt and pepper. Place the asparagus in a tinfoil sheet and fold the sides such that you create a basket. Smoke the asparagus for 1 hour or until soft turning after half an hour. Remove from the grill and serve. Enjoy.

Nutrition Info: Calories 43, Total fat 2g, Saturated fat 0g, Total Carbs 4g, Net Carbs 2g, Protein 3g, Sugar 2g, Fiber 2g, Sodium: 148mg

8. Roasted Parmesan Cheese Broccoli

Servings: 3 To 4   Cooking Time: 45 Minutes
Ingredients:
- 3cups broccoli, stems trimmed
- 1tbsp lemon juice
- 1tbsp olive oil
- 2garlic cloves, minced
- 1/2 tsp kosher salt
- 1/2 tsp ground black pepper
- 1tsp lemon zest
- 1/8 cup parmesan cheese, grated

Directions:

Preheat pellet grill to 375°F. Place broccoli in a resealable bag. Add lemon juice, olive oil, garlic cloves, salt, and pepper. Seal the bag and toss to combine. Let the mixture marinate for 30 minutes. Pour broccoli into a grill basket. Place basket on grill grates to roast. Grill broccoli for 14-18 minutes, flipping broccoli halfway through. Grill until tender yet a little crispy on the outside. Remove broccoli from grill and place on a serving dish—zest with lemon and top with grated parmesan cheese. Serve immediately and enjoy!

Nutrition Info: Calories: 82.6 Fat: 4.6 g Cholesterol: 1.8 mg Carbohydrate: 8.1 g Fiber: 4.6 g Sugar: 0 Protein: 5.5

9. Corn Chowder

Servings: 3 To 4   Cooking Time: 35 Minutes
Ingredients:
- 1/4 tsp. Cajun Seasoning
- 2tbsp. Butter, unsalted
- 2tbsp. Parsley, fresh and minced
- 1Onion quartered
- 1/2 cup Celery Stalks, diced
- 1/4 tsp. Sea Salt
- 2Garlic cloves
- 1/4 cup Heavy Cream
- 1/2 cup Carrot, diced
- 3cups Corn Kernels, frozen
- 2-1/2 cups Vegetable Broth
- 1/4 tsp. Black Pepper, grounded
- 1Red Potato, chopped

Directions:

To start with, keep butter, onion, and garlic in the pitcher of the blender. After that, press the 'saute' button. Next, stir in all the remaining ingredients to the pitcher and select the 'hearty soup' button. Once the program gets over, transfer the soup to serving bowls and serve immediately. Garnish with parsley leaves.

Nutrition Info: Calories: 499 Fat: 40 g Total Carbs: 32 g Fiber: 2.5 g Sugar: 7.3 g Protein: 6.8 g Cholesterol: 120 mg

10. Grilled Corn On The Cob With Parmesan And Garlic

Servings: 6   Cooking Time: 30 Minutes
Ingredients:
- 4 tablespoons butter, melted
- 2 cloves of garlic, minced
- Salt and pepper to taste
- 8 corns, unhusked
- ½ cup parmesan cheese, grated
- 1 tablespoon parsley chopped

Directions:

Fire the Grill to 450F. Use desired wood pellets when cooking. Close the lid and preheat for 15 minutes. Place butter, garlic, salt, and pepper in a bowl and mix until well combined. Peel the corn husk but do not detach the husk from the corn. Remove the silk. Brush the corn with the garlic butter mixture and close the husks. Place the corn on the grill grate and cook for 30 minutes turning the corn every 5 minutes for even cooking.

Nutrition Info: Calories per serving: 272; Protein: 8.8g; Carbs: 38.5g; Fat: 12.3g Sugar: 6.6g

11. Smoked Tofu

Servings: 4   Cooking Time: 41 Hour And 30 Minutes

Ingredients:
- 400g plain tofu
- Sesame oil

Directions:
Preheat the smoker to 225°F while adding wood chips and water to it.   Till that time, take the tofu out of the packet and let it rest   Slice the tofu in one-inch thick pieces and apply sesame oil   Place the tofu inside the smoker for 45 minutes while adding water and wood chips after one hour.   Once cooked, take them out and serve!

Nutrition Info: Calories: 201 Cal Fat: 13 g Carbohydrates: 1 g   Protein: 20 g Fiber: 0 g

12. Vegan Smoked Carrot Dogs

Servings: 2   Cooking Time: 35 Minutes

Ingredients:
- 4 carrots, thick
- 2 tbsp avocado oil
- 1/2 tbsp garlic powder
- 1 tbsp liquid smoke
- Pepper to taste
- Kosher salt to taste

Directions:
Preheat your   to 425F then line a parchment paper on a baking sheet.   Peel the carrots to resemble a hot dog. Round the edges when peeling.   Whisk together oil, garlic powder, liquid smoke, pepper and salt in a bowl, small.   Now place carrots on the baking sheet and pour the mixture over. Roll your carrots in the mixture to massage seasoning and oil into them. Use fingertips. Roast the carrots in the   until fork tender for about 35 minutes. Brush the carrots using the marinade mixture every 5 minutes.   Remove and place into hot dog buns then top with hot dog toppings of your choice.   Serve and enjoy!

Nutrition Info: Calories 76, Total fat 1.8g, Saturated 0.4g, Total 14.4g, Net carbs 10.6g, Protein 1.5g, Sugar 6.6g, Fiber 3.8g, Sodium 163mg, Potassium 458mg

13. Easy Smoked Vegetables

Servings: 6   Cooking Time: 1 ½ Hour

Ingredients:
- 1 cup of pecan wood chips
- 1 ear fresh corn, silk strands removed, and husks, cut corn into 1-inch pieces
- 1 medium yellow squash, 1/2-inch slices
- 1 small red onion, thin wedges
- 1 small green bell pepper, 1-inch strips
- 1 small red bell pepper, 1-inch strips
- 1 small yellow bell pepper, 1-inch strips
- 1 cup mushrooms, halved
- 2 tbsp vegetable oil
- Vegetable seasonings

Directions:

Take a large bowl and toss all the vegetables together in it. Sprinkle it with seasoning and coat all the vegetables well with it.   Place the wood chips and a bowl of water in the smoker.   Preheat the smoker at 100°F or ten minutes.   Put the vegetables in a pan and add to the middle rack of the electric smoker.   Smoke for thirty minutes until the vegetable becomes tender.   When done, serve, and enjoy.

Nutrition Info: Calories: 97 Cal Fat: 5 g Carbohydrates: 11 g   Protein: 2 g Fiber: 3 g

14. Zucchini With Red Potatoes

Servings: 4   Cooking Time: 4 Hours

Ingredients:
- 2 zucchinis, sliced in 3/4-inch-thick disks
- 1 red pepper, cut into strips
- 2 yellow squash, sliced in 3/4-inch-thick disks
- 1 medium red onion, cut into wedges
- 6 small red potatoes, cut into chunks
- Balsamic Vinaigrette:
- 1/3 cup extra virgin olive oil
- 1/4 teaspoon salt
- 1/4 cup balsamic vinegar
- 2 tsp Dijon mustard
- 1/8 teaspoon pepper

Directions:
For Vinaigrette: Take a medium-sized bowl and blend together olive oil, Dijon mustard, salt, pepper, and balsamic vinegar.   Place all the veggies into a large bowl and pour the vinaigrette mixture over it and evenly toss.   Put the vegetable in a pan and then smoke for 4 hours at a temperature of 225°F.   Serve and enjoy the food.

Nutrition Info: Calories: 381 Cal Fat: 17.6 g Carbohydrates: 49 g   Protein: 6.7 g Fiber: 6.5 g

15. Grilled Baby Carrots And Fennel

Servings: 8   Cooking Time: 30 Minutes

Ingredients:
- 1-pound slender rainbow carrots, washed and peeled
- 2 whole fennel bulbs, chopped
- 2 tablespoons extra virgin olive oil
- 1 teaspoon salt
- Salt to taste

Directions:
Fire the   Grill to 500F. Use desired wood pellets when cooking. Close the lid and preheat for 15 minutes. Place all ingredients in a sheet tray and toss to coat with oil and seasoning.   Place on the grill grate and cook for 30 minutes.

Nutrition Info: Calories per serving:52 ;
Protein: 1.2g; Carbs: 8.9g; Fat: 1.7g Sugar: 4.3g

16. Smoked Eggs

Servings: 12   Cooking Time: 30 Minutes

Ingredients:
- 12 hardboiled eggs, peeled and rinsed

Directions:
Supply your smoker with wood pellets and follow the manufacturer's specific start-up procedure. Preheat the grill, with the lid closed, to 120°F. Place the eggs directly on the grill grate and smoke for 30 minutes. They will begin to take on a slight brown sheen. Remove the eggs and refrigerate for at least 30 minutes before serving. Refrigerate any leftovers in an airtight container for 1 or 2 weeks.

17. Smoked Pumpkin Soup

Servings: 6   Cooking Time: 1 Hour And 33 Minutes

Ingredients:
- 5 pounds pumpkin, seeded and sliced
- 3 tablespoons butter
- 1 onion, diced
- 2 cloves garlic, minced
- 1 tablespoon brown sugar
- 1 teaspoon paprika
- ¼ teaspoon ground cinnamon
- ¼ teaspoon ground nutmeg
- ½ cup apple cider
- 5 cups broth
- ½ cup cream

Directions:
Fire the Grill to 180F. Use desired wood pellets when cooking. Close the lid and preheat for 15 minutes. Place the pumpkin on the grill grate and smoke for an hour or until tender. Allow to cool. Melt the butter in a large saucepan over medium heat and sauté the onion and garlic for 3 minutes. Stir in the rest of the ingredients including the smoked pumpkin. Cook for another 30 minutes. Transfer to a blender and pulse until smooth.
Nutrition Info: Calories per serving: 246; Protein: 8.8g; Carbs: 32.2g; Fat: 11.4g Sugar: 15.5g

18. Carolina Baked Beans

Servings: 12 To 15 Minutes   Cooking Time: 2 To 3 Hours

Ingredients:
- 3 (28-ounce) cans baked beans (I like Bush's brand)
- 1 large onion, finely chopped
- 1 cup The Ultimate BBQ Sauce
- ½ cup light brown sugar
- ¼ cup Worcestershire sauce
- 3 tablespoons yellow mustard
- Nonstick cooking spray or butter, for greasing
- 1 large bell pepper, cut into thin rings
- ½ pound thick-cut bacon, partially cooked and cut into quarters

Directions:
Supply your smoker with wood pellets and follow the manufacturer's specific start-up procedure. Preheat, with the lid closed, to 300°F. In a large mixing bowl, stir together the beans, onion, barbecue sauce, brown sugar, Worcestershire sauce, and mustard until well combined. Coat a 9-by-13-inch aluminum pan with cooking spray or butter. Pour the beans into the pan and top with the bell pepper rings and bacon pieces, pressing them down slightly into the sauce. Place a layer of heavy-duty foil on the grill grate to catch drips, and place the pan on top of the foil. Close the lid and cook for 2 hours 30 minutes to 3 hours, or until the beans are hot, thick, and bubbly. Let the beans rest for 5 minutes before serving.

19. Grilled Zucchini Squash Spears

Servings: 4   Cooking Time: 10 Minutes

Ingredients:
- 4 zucchini, medium
- 2 tbsp olive oil
- 1 tbsp sherry vinegar
- 2 thyme, leaves pulled
- Salt to taste
- Pepper to taste

Directions:
Clean zucchini, cut ends off, half each lengthwise, and cut each half into thirds. Combine all the other ingredients in a zip lock bag, medium, then add spears. Toss well and mix to coat the zucchini. Preheat to 350F with the lid closed for about 15 minutes. Remove spears from the zip lock bag and place them directly on your grill grate with the cut side down. Cook for about 3-4 minutes until zucchini is tender and grill marks show. Remove them from the grill and enjoy.
Nutrition Info: Calories 93, Total fat 7.4g, Saturated fat 1.1g, Total carbs 7.1g, Net carbs 4.9g, Protein 2.4g, Sugars 3.4g, Fiber 2.2g, Sodium 59mg, Potassium 515mg

20. Grilled Baby Carrots And Fennel With Romesco

Servings: 8 To 12   Cooking Time: 45 Minutes

Ingredients:
- 1 Pound Slender Rainbow Carrots
- 2 Whole Fennel, bulb
- 2 Tablespoon extra-virgin olive oil
- 1 Teaspoon salt
- 2 Tablespoon extra-virgin olive oil
- To Taste salt
- 1 Tablespoon fresh thyme

Directions:
When ready to cook, set temperature to High and preheat, lid closed for 15 minutes. For optimal results, set to 500°F if available. Trim the carrot tops to 1". Peel the carrots and halve any larger ones so they are all about 1/2" thick. Cut the fennel bulbs lengthwise into 1/2" thick slices. Place the fennel and potato slices in a large mixing bowl. Drizzle with 2 Tbsp of the olive oil and a teaspoon of salt. Toss to coat the vegetables evenly with the oil. Place the carrots on a sheet pan. Drizzle

with the additional 2 Tbsp of olive oil and a generous pinch of salt. Brush the olive oil over the carrots to distribute evenly.   Add the potatoes and fennel slices to the sheet pan. Nestle a few sprigs of herbs into the vegetables as well.   Place the pan directly on the grill grate and cook, stirring occasionally until the vegetables are browned and softened, about 35-45 minutes. Allow to cool and serve with the Smoked Romesco Sauce. Enjoy!

21. Baked Cheesy Corn Pudding

Servings: 6   Cooking Time: 30 Minutes
Ingredients:
- 3 cloves of garlic, chopped
- 3 tablespoons butter
- 3 cups whole corn kernels
- 8 ounces cream cheese
- 1 cup cheddar cheese
- 1 cup parmesan cheese
- 1 tablespoon salt
- ½ tablespoon black pepper
- ½ cup dry breadcrumbs
- 1 cup mozzarella cheese, grated
- 1 tablespoon thyme, minced

Directions:
Fire the   Grill to 350F. Use desired wood pellets when cooking. Close the lid and preheat for 15 minutes. In a large saucepan, sauté the garlic and butter for 2 minutes until fragrant. Add the corn, cheddar cheese, parmesan cheese, salt, and pepper. Heat until the corn is melted then pour into a baking dish.   In a small bowl, combine the breadcrumbs, mozzarella cheese, and thyme.   Spread the cheese and bread crumb mixture on top of the corn mixture.   Place the baking dish on the grill grate and cook for 25 minutes.   Allow to rest before removing from the mold.

Nutrition Info: Calories per serving: 523;
Protein: 29.4g; Carbs: 34g; Fat: 31.2g Sugar: 10.8g

22. Smoked Tomato And Mozzarella Dip

Servings: 4   Cooking Time: 1 Hour
Ingredients:
- 8ounces smoked mozzarella cheese, shredded
- 8ounces Colby cheese, shredded
- ½ cup parmesan cheese, grated
- 1cup sour cream
- 1cup sun-dried tomatoes
- 1and ½ teaspoon salt
- 1teaspoon fresh ground pepper
- 1teaspoon dried basil
- 1teaspoon dried oregano
- 1teaspoon red pepper flakes
- 1garlic clove, minced
- ½ teaspoon onion powder
- French toast, serving

Directions:
Preheat your smoker to 275 degrees Fahrenheit using your preferred wood   Take a large bowl and stir in the cheeses, tomatoes, pepper, salt, basil, oregano, red pepper flakes, garlic, onion powder and mix well Transfer the mix to a small metal pan and transfer to a smoker   Smoke for 1 hour   Serve with toasted French bread   Enjoy!
Nutrition Info: Calories: 174 Fats: 11g Carbs: 15g Fiber: 2g

23. Bacon-wrapped Jalapeno Poppers

Servings: 6   Cooking Time: 20 Minutes
Ingredients:
- 6 jalapenos, Fresh
- 1/2 cup shredded cheddar cheese
- 4 oz soft cream cheese
- 1-1/2 tbsp   veggie rub
- 12 bacon slices, thin cut

Directions:
Preheat your   grill to 375F.   Halve the jalapenos lengthwise then scrape membrane and seeds using a spoon. rinse them and set aside.   Meanwhile, combine cheddar cheese, cream cheese, and veggie rub in a bowl, medium stirring until incorporated fully.   Fill the jalapenos with your cheese mixture then wrap each half with a bacon slice.   Place on your grill and grill for about 15-20 minutes until bacon becomes crispy and peppers are soft.   Serve and enjoy.

Nutrition Info: Calories 329, Total fat 25.7g, Saturated fat 11.4g, Total carbs 5g, Net carbs 4.6g, Protein 18.1g, Sugars 0.6g, Fiber 0.4g, Sodium 1667mg, Potassium 277mg

24. Blt Pasta Salad

Servings: 6   Cooking Time: 35 To 45 Minutes
Ingredients:
- 1 pound thick-cut bacon
- 16 ounces bowtie pasta, cooked according to package directions and drained
- 2 tomatoes, chopped
- ½ cup chopped scallions
- ½ cup Italian dressing
- ½ cup ranch dressing
- 1 tablespoon chopped fresh basil
- 1 teaspoon salt
- 1 teaspoon freshly ground black pepper
- 1 teaspoon garlic powder
- 1 head lettuce, cored and torn

Directions:
Supply your smoker with wood pellets and follow the manufacturer's specific start-up procedure. Preheat, with the lid closed, to 225°F.   Arrange the bacon slices on the grill grate, close the lid, and cook for 30 to 45 minutes, flipping after 20 minutes, until crisp. Remove the bacon from the grill and chop.   In a large bowl, combine the chopped bacon with the cooked pasta, tomatoes, scallions, Italian dressing, ranch dressing, basil, salt, pepper, and garlic powder. Refrigerate until ready to serve.   Toss in the lettuce just before serving to keep it from wilting.

25. Grilled Artichokes

Servings: 6   Cooking Time: 15 Minutes
Ingredients:
- 3 large artichokes, blanched and halved
- 3 + 3 tablespoons olive oil
- Salt and pepper to taste
- 1 cup mayonnaise
- 1 cup yogurt
- 2 tablespoons parsley, chopped
- 2 tablespoons capers
- Lemon juice to taste

Directions:
Fire the   Grill to 500F. Use desired wood pellets when cooking. Close the lid and preheat for 15 minutes. Brush the artichokes with 3 tablespoons of olive oil. Season with salt and pepper to taste.   Place on the grill grate and cook for 15 minutes.   Allow to cool before slicing.   Once cooled, slice the artichokes and place in a bowl.   In another bowl, mix together the mayonnaise, yogurt, parsley, capers, and lemon juice. Season with salt and pepper to taste. Mix until well-combined.   Pour sauce over the artichokes.   Toss to coat.
Nutrition Info: Calories per serving: 257; Protein: 6.7g; Carbs: 13.2 g; Fat: 20.9g Sugar: 3.7g

26. Scampi Spaghetti Squash

Servings: 4   Cooking Time: 40 Minutes
Ingredients:
- 1 spaghetti squash
- 2 tablespoons extra-virgin olive oil
- 1 teaspoon salt
- 1 teaspoon freshly ground black pepper
- 2 teaspoons garlic powder
- 4 tablespoons (½ stick) unsalted butter
- ½ cup white wine
- 1 tablespoon minced garlic
- 2 teaspoons chopped fresh parsley
- 1 teaspoon red pepper flakes
- ½ teaspoon salt
- ½ teaspoon freshly ground black pepper

Directions:
For the squash: Supply your smoker with wood pellets and follow the manufacturer's specific start-up procedure. Preheat, with the lid closed, to 375°F.   Cut off both ends of the squash, then cut it in half lengthwise. Scoop out and discard the seeds.   Rub the squash flesh well with the olive oil and sprinkle on the salt, pepper, and garlic powder.   Place the squash cut-side up on the grill grate, close the lid, and smoke for 40 minutes, or until tender   For the sauce: On the stove top, in a medium saucepan over medium heat, combine the butter, white wine, minced garlic, parsley, red pepper flakes, salt, and pepper, and cook for about 5 minutes, or until heated through. Reduce the heat to low and keep the sauce warm.   Remove the squash from the grill and let cool slightly before shredding the flesh with a fork; discard the skin.   Stir the shredded squash into the garlic-wine butter sauce and serve immediately.

27. Smoked Acorn Squash

Servings: 6   Cooking Time: 2 Hours
Ingredients:
- 3 acorn squash, seeded and halved
- 3 tbsp olive oil
- 1/4 cup butter, unsalted
- 1 tbsp cinnamon, ground
- 1 tbsp chili powder
- 1 tbsp nutmeg, ground
- 1/4 cup brown sugar

Directions:
Brush the cut sides of your squash with olive oil then cover with foil poking holes for smoke and steam to get through.   Preheat your   to 225F.   Place the squash halves on the grill with the cut side down and smoke for about 1½- 2 hours. Remove from the .   Let it sit while you prepare spiced butter. Melt butter in a saucepan then add spices and sugar stirring to combine.   Remove the foil form the squash halves.   Place 1 tbsp of the butter mixture onto each half.   Serve and enjoy!
Nutrition Info: Calories 149, Total 10g, Saturated fat 5g, Total carbs 14g, Net carbs 12g, Protein 2g, Sugars 2g, Fiber 2g, Sodium 19mg, Potassium 101m

28. Southern Slaw

Servings: 10   Cooking Time: 1 Hour And 10 Minutes
Ingredients:
- 1 head cabbage, shredded
- ¼ cup white vinegar
- ¼ cup sugar
- 1 teaspoon paprika
- ½ teaspoon salt
- ½ teaspoon freshly ground black pepper
- 1 cup heavy (whipping) cream

Directions:
Place the shredded cabbage in a large bowl.   In a small bowl, combine the vinegar, sugar, paprika, salt, and pepper.   Pour the vinegar mixture over the cabbage and mix well.   Fold in the heavy cream and refrigerate for at least 1 hour before serving.

29. Smoked Mashed Red Potatoes

Servings: 8   Cooking Time: 30 Minutes
Ingredients:
- 8 large potatoes
- Salt and pepper to taste
- ½ cup heavy cream
- ¼ cup butter

Directions:
Fire the   Grill to 180F. Use desired wood pellets when cooking. Close the lid and preheat for 15 minutes. Slice the potatoes into half and season with salt and pepper to taste. Place on a baking tray.   Place the tray with the potatoes on the grill grate and cook for 30 minutes. Be sure to flip the potatoes halfway through the cooking time.   Once cooked, remove from the grill and

place on a bowl. Add the rest of the ingredients and mash until well-combined.
Nutrition Info: Calories per serving: 363 ;
Protein: 7.8g; Carbs: 65.2g; Fat: 8.9g Sugar: 3.4g

30. Roasted Vegetable Medley

Servings: 4 To 6   Cooking Time: 50 Minutes
Ingredients:
- 2medium potatoes, cut to 1 inch wedges
- 2red bell peppers, cut into 1 inch cubes
- 1small butternut squash, peeled and cubed to 1 inch cube
- 1red onion, cut to 1 inch cubes
- 1cup broccoli, trimmed
- 2tbsp olive oil
- 1tbsp balsamic vinegar
- 1tbsp fresh rosemary, minced
- 1tbsp fresh thyme, minced
- 1tsp kosher salt
- 1tsp ground black pepper

Directions:
Preheat pellet grill to 425°F.   In a large bowl, combine potatoes, peppers, squash, and onion.   In a small bowl, whisk together olive oil, balsamic vinegar, rosemary, thyme, salt, and pepper.   Pour marinade over vegetables and toss to coat. Allow resting for about 15 minutes.   Place marinated vegetables into a grill basket, and place a grill basket on the grill grate. Cook for about 30-40 minutes, occasionally tossing in the grill basket.   Remove veggies from grill and transfer to a serving dish. Allow to cool for 5 minutes, then serve and enjoy!
Nutrition Info: Calories: 158.6 Fat: 7.4 g Cholesterol: 0 Carbohydrate: 22 g Fiber: 7.2 g Sugar: 3.1 g Protein: 5.2 g

31. Apple Veggie Burger

Servings: 6   Cooking Time: 35 Minutes
Ingredients:
- 3 tbsp ground flax or ground chia
- 1/3 cup of warm water
- 1/2 cups rolled oats
- 1 cup chickpeas, drained and rinsed
- 1 tsp cumin
- 1/2 cup onion
- 1 tsp dried basil
- 2 granny smith apples
- 1/3 cup parsley or cilantro, chopped
- 2 tbsp soy sauce
- 2 tsp liquid smoke
- 2 cloves garlic, minced
- 1 tsp chili powder
- 1/4 tsp black pepper

Directions:
Preheat the smoker to 225°F while adding wood chips and water to it.   In a separate bowl, add chickpeas and mash. Mix together the remaining ingredients along with the dipped flax seeds.   Form patties from this mixture.   Put the patties on the rack of the smoker and smoke them for 20 minutes on each side.   When brown, take them out, and serve.
Nutrition Info: Calories: 241 Cal Fat: 5 g Carbohydrates: 40 g   Protein: 9 g Fiber: 10.3 g

32. Bacon-wrapped Jalapeño Poppers

Servings: 8 To 12   Cooking Time: 40 Minutes
Ingredients:
- 12 large jalapeño peppers
- 8 oz cream cheese, softened
- 1cup pepper jack cheese, shredded
- Juice of 1 lemon1/2 tsp garlic powder
- 1/4 tsp kosher salt
- 1/4 tsp ground black pepper
- 12 bacon slices, cut in half

Directions:
Preheat pellet grill to 400°F.   Slice jalapeños in half lengthwise. Remove seeds and scrape sides with a spoon to remove the membrane.   In a medium bowl, mix cream cheese, pepper jack cheese, garlic powder, salt, and pepper until thoroughly combined.   Use a spoon or knife to place the cream cheese mixture into each jalapeño half. Make sure not to fill over the sides of the jalapeño half.   Wrap each cheese-filled pepper with a half slice of bacon. If you can't get a secure wrap, then hold bacon and pepper together with a toothpick.   Place assembled poppers on the grill and cook for 15-20 minutes or until bacon is crispy.   Remove from grill, allow to cool, then serve and enjoy!
Nutrition Info: Calories: 78.8 Fat: 7.2 g Cholesterol: 19.2 mg Carbohydrate: 1 g Fiber: 0.2 g Sugar: 0.7 g Protein: 2.5 g

33. Baked Sweet And Savory Yams

Servings: 6   Cooking Time: 55 Minutes
Ingredients:
- 3 pounds yams, scrubbed
- 3 tablespoons extra virgin olive oil
- Honey to taste
- Goat cheese as needed
- ½ cup brown sugar
- ½ cup pecans, chopped

Directions:
Fire the   Grill to 350F. Use desired wood pellets when cooking. Close the lid and preheat for 15 minutes. Poke holes on the yams using a fork. Wrap yams in foil and place on the grill grate. Cook for 45 minutes until tender.   Remove the yams from the grill and allow to cool. Once cooled, peel the yam and slice to ¼" rounds. Place on a parchment-lined baking tray and brush with olive oil. Drizzle with honey, cheese, brown sugar, and pecans.   Place in the grill and cook for another 10 minutes.
Nutrition Info: Calories per serving: 421;
Protein: 4.3g; Carbs: 82.4g; Fat: 9.3g Sugar:19.3 g

34. Smoked Watermelon

Servings: 5   Cooking Time: 45-90 Minutes
Ingredients:
- 1 small seedless watermelon
- Balsamic vinegar
- Wooden skewers

Directions:
Slice ends of small seedless watermelons   Slice the watermelon in 1-inch cubes. Put the cubes in a container and drizzle vinegar on the cubes of watermelon. Preheat the smoker to 225°F. Add wood chips and water to the smoker before starting preheating.   Place the cubes on the skewers.   Place the skewers on the smoker rack for 50 minutes.   Cook   Remove the skewers.   Serve!
Nutrition Info: Calories: 20 Cal Fat: 0 g Carbohydrates: 4 g   Protein: 1 g Fiber: 0.2 g

35. Chicken Tortilla Soup

Servings: 4   Cooking Time: 35 Minutes
Ingredients:
- 1/2 cup Black Beans, canned
- 1Jalapeno Pepper, halved and seeds removed
- 1-1/2 cup Chicken Stock
- 2Carrots, sliced into ¼-inch pieces
- 1/2 of 1 Onion, peeled and halved
- 1/2 cup Corn
- 3 Garlic cloves
- 14-1/2 oz. Fire Roasted Tomatoes
- 1/4 cup Cilantro Leaves
- 10 oz. Chicken Breast, diced into ½ inch
- For the seasoning mix:
- 1/4 tsp. Chipotle
- 1tsp. Cuminutes
- 1/2 tsp. Sea Salt
- 1/2 tsp. Smoked Paprika

Directions:
Place pepper, carrots, onion, garlic cloves, and cilantro in the blender pitcher.   Pulse the mixture for 3 minutes and then pour the chicken stock to it.   Pulse again for another 3 minutes.   Next, stir in the remaining ingredients and press the 'hearty soup' button.   Finally, transfer to the serving bowl.
Nutrition Info: Calories: 260 Fat: 4 g Total Carbs: 40 g Fiber: 5.9 g Sugar: 8 g Protein: 14 g Cholesterol: 20 mg

36. Smoked Balsamic Potatoes And Carrots

Servings: 6   Cooking Time: 10 Minutes
Ingredients:
- 2 large carrots, peeled and chopped roughly
- 2 large Yukon Gold potatoes, peeled and wedged
- 5 tablespoons olive oil
- 5 tablespoons balsamic vinegar
- Salt and pepper to taste

Directions:
Fire the   Grill to 400F. Use desired wood pellets when cooking. Close the lid and preheat for 15 minutes. Place all ingredients in a bowl and toss to coat the vegetables with the seasoning.   Place on a baking tray lined with foil.   Place on the grill grate and close the lid. Cook for 30 minutes.
Nutrition Info: Calories per serving: 219; Protein: 2.9g; Carbs: 27g; Fat: 11.4g Sugar:4.5 g

37. Grilled Carrots And Asparagus

Servings: 6   Cooking Time: 30 Minutes
Ingredients:
- 1 pound whole carrots, with tops
- 1 bunch of asparagus, ends trimmed
- Sea salt as needed
- 1 teaspoon lemon zest
- 2 tablespoons honey
- 2 tablespoons olive oil

Directions:
Switch on the   grill, fill the grill hopper with flavored wood pellets, power the grill on by using the control panel, select 'smoke' on the temperature dial, or set the temperature to 450 degrees F and let it preheat for a minimum of 15 minutes.   Meanwhile, take a medium dish, place asparagus in it, season with sea salt, drizzle with oil and toss until mixed.   Take a medium bowl, place carrots in it, drizzle with honey, sprinkle with sea salt and toss until combined.   When the grill has preheated, open the lid, place asparagus and carrots on the grill grate, shut the grill and smoke for 30 minutes. When done, transfer vegetables to a dish, sprinkle with lemon zest, and then serve.
Nutrition Info: Calories: 79.8 Cal ;Fat: 4.8 g ;Carbs: 8.6 g ;Protein: 2.6 g ;Fiber: 3.5 g

38. Wood Pellet Grilled Stuffed Zucchini

Servings: 8   Cooking Time: 11 Minutes
Ingredients:
- 4 zucchini
- 5 tbsp olive oil
- 2 tbsp red onion, chopped
- 1/4 tbsp garlic, minced
- 1/2 cup bread crumbs
- 1/2 cup mozzarella cheese, shredded
- 1 tbsp fresh mint
- 1/2 tbsp salt
- 3 tbsp parmesan cheese

Directions:
Cut the zucchini lengthwise and scoop out the pulp then brush the shells with oil.   In a non-stick skillet sauté pulp, onion, and remaining oil. Add garlic and cook for a minute.   Add bread crumbs and cook until golden brown. Remove from heat and stir in mozzarella cheese, fresh mint, and salt.   Spoon the mixture into the shells and sprinkle parmesan cheese.   Place in a grill and grill for 10 minutes or until the zucchini are tender.

Nutrition Info: Calories 186, Total fat 10g, Saturated fat 5g, Total Carbs 17g, Net Carbs 14g, Protein 9g, Sugar 4g, Fiber 3g, Sodium: 553mg

39. Vegetable Sandwich

Servings: 4   Cooking Time: 45 Minutes
Ingredients:
- For the Smoked Hummus:
- 1 1/2 cups cooked chickpeas
- 1 tablespoon minced garlic
- 1 teaspoon salt
- 4 tablespoons lemon juice
- 2 tablespoon olive oil
- 1/3 cup tahini
- For the Vegetables:
- 2 large portobello mushrooms
- 1 small eggplant, destemmed, sliced into strips
- 1 teaspoon salt
- 1 small zucchini, trimmed, sliced into strips
- ½ teaspoon ground black pepper
- 1 small yellow squash, peeled, sliced into strips
- ¼ cup olive oil
- For the Cheese:
- 1 lemon, juiced
- ½ teaspoon minced garlic
- ¼ teaspoon ground black pepper
- ¼ teaspoon salt
- 1/2 cup ricotta cheese
- To Assemble:
- 1 bunch basil, leaves chopped
- 2 heirloom tomatoes, sliced
- 4 ciabatta buns, halved

Directions:
Switch on the   grill, fill the grill hopper with pecan flavored wood pellets, power the grill on by using the control panel, select 'smoke' on the temperature dial, or set the temperature to 180 degrees F and let it preheat for a minimum of 15 minutes.   Meanwhile, prepare the hummus, and for this, take a sheet tray and spread chickpeas on it.   When the grill has preheated, open the lid, place sheet tray on the grill grate, shut the grill and smoke for 20 minutes.   When done, transfer chickpeas to a food processor, add remaining ingredients for the hummus in it, and pulse for 2 minutes until smooth, set aside until required.   Change the smoking temperature to 500 degrees F, shut with lid, and let it preheat for 10 minutes.   Meanwhile, prepare vegetables and for this, take a large bowl, place all the vegetables in it, add salt and black pepper, drizzle with oil and lemon juice and toss until coated.   Place vegetables on the grill grate, shut with lid and then smoke for eggplant, zucchini, and squash for 15 minutes and mushrooms for 25 minutes.   Meanwhile, prepare the cheese and for this, take a small bowl, place all of its ingredients in it and stir until well combined. Assemble the sandwich for this, cut buns in half lengthwise, spread prepared hummus on one side, spread cheese on the other side, then stuff with grilled vegetables and top with tomatoes and basil.   Serve straight away.

Nutrition Info: Calories: 560 Cal ;Fat: 40 g ;Carbs: 45 g ;Protein: 8.3 g ;Fiber: 6.8 g

40.   Ramen Soup

Servings: 2   Cooking Time: 35 Minutes
Ingredients:
- 4cups Chicken Stock
- 1tbsp. Extra Virgin Olive Oil
- 2Baby Bok Choy Head, leaves torn
- 1Shallot, chopped into 1-inch piece
- 3oz. Ramen, dried
- 4Garlic cloves
- 1tsp. Sesame Oil, toasted
- 2tsp. Ginger, fresh
- One bunch of Green Onion, sliced thinly
- 1cup Chicken, cooked and cut into 1-inch cubes

Directions:
First, keep the olive oil, shallot, garlic, and ginger in the blender pitcher.   After that, press the 'saute' button. Next, stir in the chicken, green onions, chicken stock, and sesame oil into it.   Now, select the 'hearty soup' button. Then, three minutes before the program ends, spoon in the ramen noodles and baby bok choy.   Check the chicken's internal temperature and ensure it is 165 ° F and if it is, then transfer the soup to the serving bowls. Serve immediately and enjoy it.

Nutrition Info: Calories: 190 Fat: 8g Total Carbs: 25g Fiber: 1 g Sugar: 0.5 g Protein: 3 g Cholesterol: 2.5 mg

41.   Smoked Mushrooms

Servings: 2   Cooking Time: 45 Minutes
Ingredients:
- 4 cups whole baby portobello, cleaned
- 1 tbsp canola oil
- 1 tbsp onion powder
- 1 tbsp garlic, granulated
- 1 tbsp salt
- 1 tbsp pepper

Directions:
Place all the ingredients in a bowl, mix, and combine. Set your   to 180F.   Place the mushrooms on the grill directly and smoke for about 30 minutes.   Increase heat to high and cook the mushroom for another 15 minutes.   Serve warm and enjoy!

Nutrition Info: Calories 118, Total fat 7.6g, Saturated fat 0.6g, Total carbs 10.8g, Net carbs 8.3g, Protein 5.4g, Sugars 3.7g, Fiber 2.5g, Sodium 3500mg, Potassium 536mg

42.   Grilled Ratatouille Salad

Servings: 6   Cooking Time: 25 Minutes
Ingredients:
- 1 Whole sweet potatoes
- 1 Whole red onion, diced
- 1 Whole zucchini
- 1 Whole Squash

- 1 Large Tomato, diced
- As Needed vegetable oil
- As Needed salt and pepper

Directions:
Preheat grill to high setting with the lid closed for 10-15 minutes.   Slice all vegetables to a ¼ inch thickness. Lightly brush each vegetable with oil and season with 's Veggie Shake or salt and pepper.   Place sweet potato, onion, zucchini, and squash on grill grate and grill for 20 minutes or until tender, turn halfway through.   Add tomato slices to the grill during the last 5 minutes of cooking time.   For presentation, alternate vegetables while layering them vertically. Enjoy!

43. Vegetable Skewers

Servings: 4   Cooking Time: 20 Minutes
Ingredients:
- 2 cups whole white mushrooms
- 2 large yellow squash, peeled, chopped
- 1 cup chopped pineapple
- 1 cup chopped red pepper
- 1 cup halved strawberries
- 2 large zucchini, chopped
- For the Dressing:
- 2 lemons, juiced
- ½ teaspoon ground black pepper
- 1/2 teaspoon sea salt
- 1 teaspoon red chili powder
- 1 tablespoon maple syrup
- 1 tablespoon orange zest
- 2 tablespoons apple cider vinegar
- 1/4 cup olive oil

Directions:
Switch on the   grill, fill the grill hopper with flavored wood pellets, power the grill on by using the control panel, select 'smoke' on the temperature dial, or set the temperature to 450 degrees F and let it preheat for a minimum of 5 minutes.   Meanwhile, prepared thread vegetables and fruits on skewers alternately and then brush skewers with oil.   When the grill has preheated, open the lid, place vegetable skewers on the grill grate, shut the grill, and smoke for 20 minutes until tender and lightly charred.   Meanwhile, prepare the dressing and for this, take a small bowl, place all of its ingredients in it and then whisk until combined.   When done, transfer skewers to a dish, top with prepared dressing and then serve.
Nutrition Info: Calories: 130 Cal ;Fat: 2 g ;Carbs: 20 g ;Protein: 2 g ;Fiber: 0.3 g

44. Grilled Zucchini

Servings: 6   Cooking Time: 10 Minutes
Ingredients:
- 4 medium zucchini
- 2 tablespoons olive oil
- 1 tablespoon sherry vinegar
- 2 sprigs of thyme, leaves chopped
- ½ teaspoon salt

- 1/3 teaspoon ground black pepper

Directions:
Switch on the   grill, fill the grill hopper with oak flavored wood pellets, power the grill on by using the control panel, select 'smoke' on the temperature dial, or set the temperature to 350 degrees F and let it preheat for a minimum of 5 minutes.   Meanwhile, cut the ends of each zucchini, cut each in half and then into thirds and place in a plastic bag.   Add remaining ingredients, seal the bag, and shake well to coat zucchini pieces.   When the grill has preheated, open the lid, place zucchini on the grill grate, shut the grill and smoke for 4 minutes per side. When done, transfer zucchini to a dish, garnish with more thyme and then serve.
Nutrition Info: Calories: 74 Cal ;Fat: 5.4 g ;Carbs: 6.1 g ;Protein: 2.6 g ;Fiber: 2.3 g

45. Grilled Cherry Tomato Skewers

Servings: 4   Cooking Time: 50 Minutes
Ingredients:
- 24 cherry tomatoes
- 1/4 cup olive oil
- 3tbsp balsamic vinegar
- 4garlic cloves, minced
- 1tbsp fresh thyme, finely chopped
- 1tsp kosher salt
- 1tsp ground black pepper
- 2tbsp chives, finely chopped

Directions:
Preheat pellet grill to 425°F.   In a medium-sized bowl, mix olive oil, balsamic vinegar, garlic, and thyme. Add tomatoes and toss to coat.   Let tomatoes sit in the marinade at room temperature for about 30 minutes.   Remove tomatoes from marinade and thread 4 tomatoes per skewer.   Season both sides of each skewer with kosher salt and ground pepper.   Place on grill grate and grill for about 3 minutes on each side, or until each side is slightly charred.   Remove from grill and allow to rest for about 5 minutes. Garnish with chives, then serve and enjoy!
Nutrition Info: Calories: 228 Fat: 10 g Cholesterol: 70 mg Carbohydrate: 7 g Fiber: 2 g Sugar: 3 g Protein: 27 g

46. Smoked Pickles

Servings: 6   Cooking Time: 15 Minutes
Ingredients:
- 1-quart water
- ¼ cup sugar
- ½ quart white vinegar
- ½ cup salt
- ½ teaspoon peppercorns
- 1 ½ teaspoons celery seeds
- 1 ½ teaspoons coriander seeds
- 1 teaspoon mustard seeds
- 8 cloves of garlic, minced
- 1 bunch dill weed
- 12 small cucumbers

Directions:
Place the water, sugar, vinegar, salt, and peppercorns in a saucepan. Bring to a boil over medium flame. Transfer to a bowl and allow to cool. Add in the rest of the ingredients. Allow the cucumber to soak in the brine for at least 3 days. When ready to cook, fire the Grill to 500F. Use desired wood pellets when cooking. Close the lid and preheat for 15 minutes. Pat dry the cucumber with paper towel and place on the grill grate. Smoke for 15 minutes.
Nutrition Info: Calories per serving: 67;
Protein: 2.4g; Carbs: 12.9g; Fat: 1.1g Sugar:8.5 g

47. Roasted Butternut Squash

Servings: 4   Cooking Time: 30 Minutes
Ingredients:
- 2-pound butternut squash
- 3 tablespoon extra-virgin olive oil
- Veggie Rub, as needed

Directions:
Fire the Grill to 350F. Use desired wood pellets when cooking. Close the lid and preheat for 15 minutes. Slice the butternut squash into ½ inch thick and remove the seeds. Season with oil and veggie rub. Place the seasoned squash in a baking tray. Grill for 30 minutes.
Nutrition Info: Calories per serving: 131;
Protein: 1.9g; Carbs: 23.6g; Fat: 4.7g Sugar: 0g

48. Salt-crusted Baked Potatoes

Servings: 6   Cooking Time: 40 Minutes
Ingredients:
- 6 russet potatoes, scrubbed and dried
- 3 tablespoons oil
- 1 tablespoons salt
- Butter as needed
- Sour cream as needed

Directions:
Fire the Grill to 400F. Use desired wood pellets when cooking. Close the lid and preheat for 15 minutes. In a large bowl, coat the potatoes with oil and salt. Place seasoned potatoes on a baking tray. Place the tray with potatoes on the grill grate. Close the lid and grill for 40 minutes. Serve with butter and sour cream.
Nutrition Info: Calories per serving: 363;
Protein: 8g; Carbs: 66.8g; Fat: 8.6g Sugar: 2.3g

49. Potato Fries With Chipotle Peppers

Servings: 4   Cooking Time: 30 Minutes
Ingredients:
- 4 potatoes, sliced into strips
- 3 tablespoons olive oil
- Salt and pepper to taste
- 1 cup mayonnaise
- 2 chipotle peppers in adobo sauce
- 2 tablespoons lime juice

Directions:

Set the wood pellet grill to high. Preheat it for 15 minutes while the lid is closed. Coat the potato strips with oil. Sprinkle with salt and pepper. Put a baking pan on the grate. Transfer potato strips to the pan. Cook potatoes until crispy. Mix the remaining ingredients. Pulse in a food processor until pureed. Serve potato fries with chipotle dip. Tips: You can also use sweet potatoes instead of potatoes.

50. Wood Pellet Smoked Mushrooms

Servings: 5   Cooking Time: 45 Minutes
Ingredients:
- 4 cup portobello, whole and cleaned
- 1 tbsp canola oil
- 1 tbsp onion powder
- 1 tbsp granulated garlic
- 1tbsp salt
- 1 tbsp pepper

Directions:
In a mixing bowl, add all the ingredients and mix well. Set the wood pellet temperature to 180°F then place the mushrooms directly on the grill. Smoke the mushrooms for 30 minutes. Increase the temperature to high and cook the mushrooms for a further 15 minutes. Serve and enjoy.
Nutrition Info: Calories 1680, Total fat 30g, Saturated fat 2g, Total Carbs 10g, Net Carbs 10g, Protein 4g, Sugar 0g, Fiber 0g, Sodium: 514mg, Potassium 0mg

51. Sweet Potato Fries

Servings: 4   Cooking Time: 40 Minutes
Ingredients:
- 3 sweet potatoes, sliced into strips
- 4 tablespoons olive oil
- 2 tablespoons fresh rosemary, chopped
- Salt and pepper to taste

Directions:
Set the wood pellet grill to 450 degrees F. Preheat it for 10 minutes. Spread the sweet potato strips in the baking pan. Toss in olive oil and sprinkle with rosemary, salt and pepper. Cook for 15 minutes. Flip and cook for another 15 minutes. Flip and cook for 10 more minutes. Tips: Soak sweet potatoes in water before cooking to prevent browning.

52. Fries With Chipotle Ketchup

Servings: 6   Cooking Time: 10 Minutes
Ingredients:
- 6 Yukon Gold potatoes, scrubbed and cut into thick strips
- 1 tablespoon   Beef Rub
- 1 tablespoon extra-virgin olive oil
- 1 teaspoon onion powder
- 1 teaspoon garlic powder
- ½ cup chipotle peppers, chopped
- 1 cup ketchup

- 1 tablespoon sugar
- 1 tablespoon cumin
- 1 tablespoon chili powder
- 1 whole lime
- 2 tablespoons butter

Directions:
Place the potatoes in a bowl and stir in the Beef Rub, olive oil, onion powder, and garlic powder. Toss to coat the potatoes with the spices. Fire the Grill to 500F. Use desired wood pellets when cooking. Close the lid and preheat for 15 minutes. Place the potatoes on a baking sheet lined with foil. Place on the grill grate and cook for 10 minutes. Meanwhile, place the rest of the ingredients in a small bowl and mix until well-combined. Serve the fries with the chipotle ketchup sauce.

Nutrition Info: Calories per serving: 387 ; Protein: 8.6g; Carbs: 79.3g; Fat: 5.6g Sugar: 13.7g

53. Smoked Stuffed Mushrooms

Servings: 12   Cooking Time: 1 Hour 15 Minutes
Ingredients:
- 12-16 white mushrooms, large, cleaned and stems removed
- 1/2 cup parmesan cheese
- 1/2 cup bread crumbs, Italian
- 2 minced garlic cloves
- 2 tbsp fresh parsley, chopped
- 1/4 -1/3 cup olive oil
- Salt and pepper to taste

Directions:
Preheat your 375F. Remove mushroom very bottom stem then dice the rest into small pieces. Combine mushroom stems, parmesan cheese, bread crumbs, garlic, parsley, 3 tbsp oil, pepper, and salt in a bowl, large. Combine until moist. Layer mushrooms in a pan, disposable, then fill them with the mixture until heaping. Drizzle with more oil. Place the pan on the grill. Smoke for about 1 hour 20 minutes until filling browns and mushrooms become tender. Remove from and serve. Enjoy!

Nutrition Info: Calories 74, Total fat 6.1g, Saturated fat 1g, Total carbs 4.1g, Net carbs 3.7g, Protein 1.6g, Sugars 0.6g, Fiber 0.4g, Sodium 57mg, Potassium 72mg

54. Bunny Dogs With Sweet And Spicy Jalapeño Relish

Servings: 8   Cooking Time: 35 To 40 Minutes
Ingredients:
- 8 hot dog-size carrots, peeled
- ¼ cup honey
- ¼ cup yellow mustard
- Nonstick cooking spray or butter, for greasing
- Salt
- Freshly ground black pepper
- 8 hot dog buns
- Sweet and Spicy Jalapeño Relish

Directions:

Prepare the carrots by removing the stems and slicing in half lengthwise. In a small bowl, whisk together the honey and mustard. Supply your smoker with wood pellets and follow the manufacturer's specific start-up procedure. Preheat, with the lid closed, to 375°F. Line a baking sheet with aluminum foil and coat with cooking spray. Brush the carrots on both sides with the honey mustard and season with salt and pepper; put on the baking sheet. Place the baking sheet on the grill grate, close the lid, and smoke for 35 to 40 minutes, or until tender and starting to brown. To serve, lightly toast the hot dog buns on the grill and top each with two slices of carrot and some relish.

55. Smoked Brussels Sprouts

Servings: 6   Cooking Time: 45 Minutes
Ingredients:
- 1-1/2 pounds Brussels sprouts
- 2 cloves of garlic minced
- 2 tbsp extra virgin olive oil
- Sea salt and cracked black pepper

Directions:
Rinse sprouts Remove the outer leaves and brown bottoms off the sprouts. Place sprouts in a large bowl then coat with olive oil. Add a coat of garlic, salt, and pepper and transfer them to the pan. Add to the top rack of the smoker with water and woodchips. Smoke for 45 minutes or until reaches 250°F temperature. Serve

Nutrition Info: Calories: 84 Cal Fat: 4.9 g Carbohydrates: 7.2 g Protein: 2.6 g Fiber: 2.9 g

56. Grilled Corn With Honey Butter

Servings: 6   Cooking Time: 10 Minutes
Ingredients:
- 6 pieces corn, husked
- 2 tablespoons olive oil
- Salt and pepper to taste
- ½ cup butter, room temperature
- ½ cup honey

Directions:
Fire the Grill to 350F. Use desired wood pellets when cooking. Close the lid and preheat for 15 minutes. Brush the corn with oil and season with salt and pepper to taste. Place the corn on the grill grate and cook for 10 minutes. Make sure to flip the corn halfway through the cooking time for even cooking. Meanwhile, mix the butter and honey on a small bowl. Set aside. Once the corn is cooked, remove from the grill and brush with the honey butter sauce.

Nutrition Info: Calories per serving: 387; Protein: 5g; Carbs: 51.2g; Fat: 21.6g Sugar: 28.2g

57. Wood Pellet Bacon Wrapped Jalapeno Poppers

Servings: 6   Cooking Time: 20 Minutes

Ingredients:
- 6 jalapenos, fresh
- 4 oz cream cheese
- 1/2 cup cheddar cheese, shredded
- 1 tbsp vegetable rub
- 12 slices cut bacon

Directions:
Preheat the wood pellet smoker and grill to375°F. Slice the jalapenos lengthwise and scrape the seed and membrane. Rinse them with water and set aside.   In a mixing bowl, mix cream cheese, cheddar cheese, vegetable rub until well mixed.   Fill the jalapeno halves with the mixture then wrap with the bacon pieces. Smoke for 20 minutes or until the bacon crispy.   Serve and enjoy.

Nutrition Info: Calories 1830, Total fat 11g, Saturated fat 6g, Total Carbs 5g, Net Carbs 4g, Protein 6g, Sugar 4g, Fiber 1g

58. Grilled Vegetables

Servings: 12   Cooking Time: 15 Minutes
Ingredients:
- 1 veggie tray
- 1/4 cup vegetable oil
- 1-2 tbsp   veggie seasoning

Directions:
Preheat your to 375F.   Meanwhile, toss the veggies in oil placed on a sheet pan, large, then splash with the seasoning.   Place on the and grill for about 10-15 minutes.   Remove, serve, and enjoy.

Nutrition Info: Calories 44, Total fat 5g, Saturated fat 0g, Total carbs 1g, Net carbs 1g, Protein 0g, Sugars 0g, Fiber 0g, Sodium 36mg, Potassium 116mg

59. Smoked Mushrooms

Servings: 6   Cooking Time: 10 Minutes
Ingredients:
- 4 cups   baby portobello, whole and cleaned
- 1 tablespoon canola oil
- 1 teaspoon onion powder
- 1 teaspoon garlic powder
- Salt and pepper to taste

Directions:
Place all ingredients in a bowl and toss to coat the mushrooms with the seasoning.   Fire the   Grill to 350F. Use desired wood pellets when cooking. Close the lid and preheat for 15 minutes.   Place mushrooms on the grill grate and smoke for 10 minutes. Make sure to flip the mushrooms halfway through the cooking time. Remove from the grill and serve.

Nutrition Info: Calories per serving: 62;
Protein: 5.2g; Carbs: 6.6g; Fat: 2.9g Sugar: 0.3g

60. Feisty Roasted Cauliflower

Servings: 4   Cooking Time: 10 Minutes
Ingredients:

- 1 cauliflower head, cut into florets
- 1 tablespoon oil
- 1 cup parmesan, grated
- 2 garlic cloves, crushed
- ½ teaspoon pepper
- ½ teaspoon salt
- ¼ teaspoon paprika

Directions:
Preheat your Smoker to 180 degrees F   Transfer florets to smoker and smoke for 1 hour   Take a bowl and add all ingredients except cheese   Once smoking is done, remove florets   Increase temperature to 450 degrees F, brush florets with the brush and transfer to grill   Smoke for 10 minutes more   Sprinkle cheese on top and let them sit (Lid closed) until cheese melts   Serve and enjoy!

Nutrition Info: Calories: 45 Fats: 2g Carbs: 7g Fiber: 1g

61. Roasted Veggies & Hummus

Servings: 4   Cooking Time: 20 Minutes
Ingredients:
- 1 white onion, sliced into wedges
- 2 cups butternut squash
- 2 cups cauliflower, sliced into florets
- 1 cup mushroom buttons
- Olive oil
- Salt and pepper to taste
- Hummus

Directions:
Set the   wood pellet grill to high.   Preheat it for 10 minutes while the lid is closed.   Add the veggies to a baking pan.   Roast for 20 minutes.   Serve roasted veggies with hummus.   Tips: You can also spread a little hummus on the vegetables before roasting.

62. Zucchini Soup

Servings: 4   Cooking Time: 35 Minutes
Ingredients:
- 2 tbsp. Olive Oil
- 1lb. Zucchini, chopped coarsely
- 1 Onion quartered
- 8 oz. Watercress, chopped
- Salt and Black Pepper, as needed
- Pinch of Saffron
- 3 cups Chicken Broth
- 1 tbsp. Heavy Cream

Directions:
First, place olive oil and onion in the blender pitcher and press the 'saute' button.   Once sautéed, add all the remaining ingredients to it.   Now, press the 'smooth soup' button.   Finally, transfer the soup to the serving bowls and serve immediately.

Nutrition Info: Calories: 249 Fat: 20 g Total Carbs: 15 g Fiber: 4.1 g Sugar: 10 g Protein: 4.9 g Cholesterol: 15 mg

63. Wood Pellet Grilled Asparagus And Honey Glazed Carrots

Servings: 5   Cooking Time: 35 Minutes
Ingredients:
- 1 bunch asparagus, trimmed ends
- 1 lb carrots, peeled
- 2 tbsp olive oil
- Sea salt to taste
- 2 tbsp honey
- Lemon zest

Directions:
Sprinkle the asparagus with oil and sea salt. Drizzle the carrots with honey and salt.   Preheat the wood pellet to 165°F wit the lid closed for 15 minutes.   Place the carrots in the wood pellet and cook for 15 minutes. Add asparagus and cook for 20 more minutes or until cooked through.   Top the carrots and asparagus with lemon zest. Enjoy.
Nutrition Info: Calories 1680, Total fat 30g, Saturated fat 2g, Total Carbs 10g, Net Carbs 10g, Protein 4g, Sugar 0g, Fiber 0g, Sodium: 514mg, Potassium 0mg

64. Smoked Hummus

Servings: 6   Cooking Time: 20 Minutes
Ingredients:
- 1 ½ cups chickpeas, rinsed and drained
- ¼ cup tahini
- 1 tablespoon garlic, minced
- 2 tablespoons extra virgin olive oil
- 1 teaspoon salt
- 4 tablespoons lemon juice

Directions:
Fire the   Grill to 350F. Use desired wood pellets when cooking. Close the lid and preheat for 15 minutes. Spread the chickpeas on a sheet tray and place on the grill grate. Smoke for 20 minutes.   Let the chickpeas cool at room temperature.   Place smoked chickpeas in a blender or food processor. Add in the rest of the ingredients. Pulse until smooth.   Serve with roasted vegetables if desired.
Nutrition Info: Calories per serving: 271;
Protein: 12.1g; Carbs: 34.8g; Fat: 10.4g Sugar: 5.7g

65. Grilled Corn With Honey & Butter

Servings: 4   Cooking Time: 10 Minutes
Ingredients:
- 6 pieces corn
- 2 tablespoons olive oil
- 1/2 cup butter
- 1/2 cup honey
- 1 tablespoon smoked salt
- Pepper to taste

Directions:
Preheat the wood pellet grill to high for 15 minutes while the lid is closed.   Brush the corn with oil and butter. Grill the corn for 10 minutes, turning from time to time.

Mix honey and butter.   Brush corn with this mixture and sprinkle with smoked salt and pepper.   Tips: Slice off the kernels and serve as side dish to a main course.

66. Roasted Okra

Servings: 4   Cooking Time: 30 Minutes
Ingredients:
- Nonstick cooking spray or butter, for greasing
- 1 pound whole okra
- 2 tablespoons extra-virgin olive oil
- 2 teaspoons seasoned salt
- 2 teaspoons freshly ground black pepper

Directions:
Supply your smoker with wood pellets and follow the manufacturer's specific start-up procedure. Preheat, with the lid closed, to 400°F. Alternatively, preheat your oven to 400°F.   Line a shallow rimmed baking pan with aluminum foil and coat with cooking spray. Arrange the okra on the pan in a single layer. Drizzle with the olive oil, turning to coat. Season on all sides with the salt and pepper.   Place the baking pan on the grill grate, close the lid, and smoke for 30 minutes, or until crisp and slightly charred. Alternatively, roast in the oven for 30 minutes.   Serve hot.

67. Smoked Baked Kale Chips

Servings: 4   Cooking Time: 30 Minutes
Ingredients:
- 2 bunches kale, stems removed
- Olive oil as needed
- Salt and pepper to taste

Directions:
Fire the   Grill to 350F. Use desired wood pellets when cooking. Close the lid and preheat for 15 minutes. Place all ingredients in a bowl and toss to coat the kale with oil.   Place on a baking tray and spread the leaves evenly on all surface.   Place in the grill and cook for 30 minutes or until the kale leaves become crispy.
Nutrition Info: Calories per serving: 206 ;
Protein: 9.9g; Carbs: 21g; Fat: 12g Sugar: 0g

68. Grilled Potato Salad

Servings: 8   Cooking Time: 10 Minutes
Ingredients:
- 1 ½ pound fingerling potatoes, halved lengthwise
- 1 small jalapeno, sliced
- 10 scallions
- 2 teaspoons salt
- 2 tablespoons rice vinegar
- 2 teaspoons lemon juice
- 2/3 cup olive oil, divided

Directions:
Switch on the   grill, fill the grill hopper with pecan flavored wood pellets, power the grill on by using the control panel, select 'smoke' on the temperature dial, or set the temperature to 450 degrees F and let it preheat

for a minimum of 5 minutes. Meanwhile, prepare scallions, and for this, brush them with some oil. When the grill has preheated, open the lid, place scallions on the grill grate, shut the grill and smoke for 3 minutes until lightly charred. Then transfer scallions to a cutting board, let them cool for 5 minutes, then cut into slices and set aside until required. Brush potatoes with some oil, season with some salt and black pepper, place potatoes on the grill grate, shut the grill and smoke for 5 minutes until thoroughly cooked. Then take a large bowl, pour in remaining oil, add salt, lemon juice, and vinegar and stir until combined. Add grilled scallion and potatoes, toss until well mixed, taste to adjust seasoning and then serve.

Nutrition Info: Calories: 223.7 Cal ;Fat: 12 g ;Carbs: 27 g ;Protein: 1.9 g ;Fiber: 3.3 g

69. Caldereta Stew

Servings: 12   Cooking Time: 4 Hours
Ingredients:
- 2lb. chuck roast, sliced into cubes
- 2tablespoons olive oil
- 1carrot, sliced into cubes
- 2potatoes, sliced into cubes
- 4garlic cloves, chopped
- 2tablespoons tomato paste
- 2cups tomato sauce
- 2red bell peppers, sliced into strips
- 2green bell peppers, sliced into strips
- 2cups of water
- 1/2 cup cheddar cheese, grated
- 1/4 cup liver spread
- Salt to taste

Directions:
Put the beef in a cast iron pan. Place this in the smoking cabinet. Open the side dampers and sear slide. Set the temperature to 375 degrees F. Smoke the beef for 1 hour and 30 minutes. Flip the beef and smoke for another 1 hour and 30 minutes. Add a Dutch oven on top of the grill. Pour in the olive oil. Add the carrots and potatoes. Cook for 5 minutes. Stir in the garlic and cook for 1 minute. Transfer the beef to the Dutch oven. Stir in the tomato paste, tomato sauce, bell peppers, and water. Bring to a boil. Reduce temperature to 275 degrees F. Simmer for 1 hour. Add the cheese and liver. Season with the salt.

Nutrition Info: Calories: 191.1 Fat: 9.3 g Cholesterol: 34 mg Carbohydrates: 15.4 g Fiber: 1.8 g Sugars: 1.3 g Protein: 11.3 g

70. Smoked And Smashed New Potatoes

Servings: 4   Cooking Time: 8 Hours
Ingredients:
- 1-1/2 pounds small new red potatoes or fingerlings
- Extra virgin olive oil
- Sea salt and black pepper

- 2 tbsp softened butter

Directions:
Let the potatoes dry. Once dried, put in a pan and coat with salt, pepper, and extra virgin olive oil. Place the potatoes on the topmost rack of the smoker. Smoke for 60 minutes. Once done, take them out and smash each one   Mix with butter and season

Nutrition Info: Calories: 258 Cal Fat: 2.0 g Carbohydrates: 15.5 g   Protein: 4.1 g Fiber: 1.5 g

71. Stuffed Grilled Zucchini

Servings: 4   Cooking Time: 10 Minutes
Ingredients:
- 4 zucchini, medium
- 5 tbsp olive oil, divided
- 2 tbsp red onion, finely chopped
- 1/4 tbsp garlic, minced
- 1/2 cup bread crumbs, dry
- 1/2 cup shredded mozzarella cheese, part-skim
- 1/2 tbsp salt
- 1 tbsp fresh mint, minced
- 3 tbsp parmesan cheese, grated

Directions:
Halve zucchini lengthwise and scoop pulp ou. Leave 1/4 -inch shell. Now brush using 2 tbsp oil, set aside, and chop the pulp. Saute onion and pulp in a skillet, large, then add garlic and cook for about 1 minute. Add bread crumbs and cook while stirring for about 2 minutes until golden brown. Remove everything from heat then stir in mozzarella cheese, salt, and mint. Scoop into the zucchini shells and splash with parmesan cheese. Preheat your to 375F. Place stuffed zucchini on the grill and grill while covered for about 8-10 minutes until tender. Serve warm and enjoy.

Nutrition Info: Calories 186, Total fat 10g, Saturated fat 3g, Total carbs 17g, Net carbs 14g, Protein 9g, Sugars 4g, Fiber 3g, Sodium 553mg, Potassium 237mg

72. Grilled Scallions

Servings: 6   Cooking Time: 20 Minutes
Ingredients:
- 10 whole scallions, chopped
- ¼ cup olive oil
- Salt and pepper to taste
- 2 tablespoons rice vinegar
- 1 whole jalapeno, sliced into rings

Directions:
Fire the   Grill to 500F. Use desired wood pellets when cooking. Close the lid and preheat for 15 minutes. Place on a bowl all ingredients and toss to coat. Transfer to a parchment-lined baking tray. Place on the grill grate and cook for 20 minutes or until the scallions char.

Nutrition Info: Calories per serving: 135; Protein: 2.2 g; Carbs: 9.7 g; Fat: 10.1g Sugar: 4.6g

73. Grilled Sugar Snap Peas

Servings: 4   Cooking Time: 10 Minutes
Ingredients:
- 2-pound sugar snap peas, ends trimmed
- ½ teaspoon garlic powder
- 1 teaspoon salt
- 2/3 teaspoon ground black pepper
- 2 tablespoons olive oil

Directions:
Switch on the   grill, fill the grill hopper with apple-flavored wood pellets, power the grill on by using the control panel, select 'smoke' on the temperature dial, or set the temperature to 450 degrees F and let it preheat for a minimum of 15 minutes.   Meanwhile, take a medium bowl, place peas in it, add garlic powder and oil, season with salt and black pepper, toss until mixed and then spread on the sheet pan.   When the grill has preheated, open the lid, place the prepared sheet pan on the grill grate, shut the grill and smoke for 10 minutes until slightly charred.   Serve straight away.
Nutrition Info: Calories: 91 Cal ;Fat: 5 g ;Carbs: 9 g ;Protein: 4 g ;Fiber: 3 g

74. Spinach Soup

Servings: 4   Cooking Time: 35 Minutes
Ingredients:
- 2cups Chicken Stock
- 2tbsp. Vegetable Oil
- 1Onion quartered
- 2 ½ cup Spinach
- ½ lb. Red Potatoes, sliced thinly
- 2cups Milk, whole
- 1Leek, large and sliced thinly
- Black Pepper and Sea Salt, as needed
- 1Thyme Sprigs
- 1Bay Leaf

Directions:
For making this healthy soup, place the oil, onion, bay leaf, and thyme in the blender pitcher.   Now, press the 'saute' button.   Once sautéed, stir in the rest of the ingredients and press the 'smooth soup' button. Finally, transfer the soup to the serving bowls and serve it hot.
Nutrition Info: Calories: 403 Fat: 24 g Total Carbs: 32 g Fiber: 3 g Sugar: 5.5 g Protein: 15 g Cholesterol: 66 mg

75. Broccoli-cauliflower Salad

Servings: 4   Cooking Time: 25 Minutes
Ingredients:
- 1½ cups mayonnaise
- ½ cup sour cream
- ¼ cup sugar
- 1 bunch broccoli, cut into small pieces
- 1 head cauliflower, cut into small pieces
- 1 small red onion, chopped
- 6 slices bacon, cooked and crumbled (precooked bacon works well)
- 1 cup shredded Cheddar cheese

Directions:
In a small bowl, whisk together the mayonnaise, sour cream, and sugar to make a dressing.   In a large bowl, combine the broccoli, cauliflower, onion, bacon, and Cheddar cheese.   Pour the dressing over the vegetable mixture and toss well to coat.   Serve the salad chilled.

76. Smokey Roasted Cauliflower

Servings: 4 To 6   Cooking Time: 1 Hour 20 Minutes
Ingredients:
- 1head cauliflower
- cup parmesan cheese
- Spice Ingredients:
- 1tbsp olive oil
- 2cloves garlic, chopped
- 1tsp kosher salt
- 1tsp smoked paprika

Directions:
Preheat pellet grill to 180°F. If applicable, set smoke setting to high.   Cut cauliflower into bite-size flowerets and place in a grill basket. Place basket on the grill grate and smoke for an hour.   Mix spice Ingredients In a small bowl while the cauliflower is smoking. Remove cauliflower from the grill after an hour and let cool.   Change grill temperature to 425°F. After the cauliflower has cooled, put cauliflower in a resealable bag, and pour marinade in the bag. Toss to combine in the bag.   Place cauliflower back in a grill basket and return to grill. Roast in the grill basket for 10-12 minutes or until the outsides begin to get crispy and golden brown.   Remove from grill and transfer to a serving dish. Sprinkle parmesan cheese over the cauliflower and rest for a few minutes so the cheese can melt. Serve and enjoy!
Nutrition Info: Calories: 70 Fat: 35 g Cholesterol: 0 Carbohydrate: 7 g Fiber: 3 g Sugar: 3 g Protein: 3 g

77. Baked Parmesan Mushrooms

Servings: 8   Cooking Time: 15 Minutes
Ingredients:
- 8 mushroom caps
- 1/2 cup Parmesan cheese, grated
- 1/2 teaspoon garlic salt
- 1/4 cup mayonnaise
- Pinch paprika
- Hot sauce

Directions:
Place mushroom caps in a baking pan.   Mix the remaining ingredients in a bowl.   Scoop the mixture onto the mushroom.   Place the baking pan on the grill. Cook in the   wood pellet grill at 350 degrees F for 15 minutes while the lid is closed.   Tips: You can also add chopped sausage to the mixture.

78. Green Beans With Bacon

Servings: 6   Cooking Time: 20 Minutes
Ingredients:
- 4 strips of bacon, chopped
- 1 1/2 pound green beans, ends trimmed
- 1 teaspoon minced garlic
- 1 teaspoon salt
- 4 tablespoons olive oil

Directions:
Switch on the   grill, fill the grill hopper with flavored wood pellets, power the grill on by using the control panel, select 'smoke' on the temperature dial, or set the temperature to 450 degrees F and let it preheat for a minimum of 15 minutes.   Meanwhile, take a sheet tray, place all the ingredients in it and toss until mixed. When the grill has preheated, open the lid, place prepared sheet tray on the grill grate, shut the grill and smoke for 20 minutes until lightly browned and cooked. When done, transfer green beans to a dish and then serve.
Nutrition Info: Calories: 93 Cal ;Fat: 4.6 g ;Carbs: 8.2 g ;Protein: 5.9 g ;Fiber: 2.9 g

79. Smoked Baked Beans

Servings: 12   Cooking Time: 3 Hours
Ingredients:
- 1 medium yellow onion diced
- 3 jalapenos
- 56 oz pork and beans
- 3/4 cup barbeque sauce
- 1/2 cup dark brown sugar
- 1/4 cup apple cider vinegar
- 2 tbsp Dijon mustard
- 2 tbsp molasses

Directions:
Preheat the smoker to 250°F. Pour the beans along with all the liquid in a pan. Add brown sugar, barbeque sauce, Dijon mustard, apple cider vinegar, and molasses. Stir. Place the pan on one of the racks. Smoke for 3 hours until thickened. Remove after 3 hours. Serve
Nutrition Info: Calories: 214 Cal Fat: 2 g
Carbohydrates: 42 g   Protein: 7 g Fiber: 7 g

80. Grilled Broccoli

Servings: 1-2   Cooking Time: 3 Minutes
Ingredients:
- 2cups of broccoli, fresh
- 1tablespoon of canola oil
- 1teaspoon of lemon pepper

Directions:
Place the grill; grate inside the unit and close the hood. Preheat the grill by turning at high for 10 minutes. Meanwhile, mix broccoli with lemon pepper and canola oil.   Toss well to coat the Ingredients: thoroughly. Place it on a grill grade once add food appears.   Lock the unit and cook for 3 minutes at medium.   Take out and serve.

Nutrition Info: Calories: 96 Total Fat: 7.3g Saturated Fat: 0.5g Cholesterol: 0mg Sodium: 30mg Total Carbohydrate: 6.7g Dietary Fiber 2.7g Total Sugars: 1.6g Protein: 2.7g

81. Grilled Sweet Potato Planks

Servings: 8   Cooking Time: 30 Minutes
Ingredients:
- 5 sweet potatoes, sliced into planks
- 1 tablespoon olive oil
- 1 teaspoon onion powder
- Salt and pepper to taste

Directions:
Set the   wood pellet grill to high.   Preheat it for 15 minutes while the lid is closed.   Coat the sweet potatoes with oil.   Sprinkle with onion powder, salt and pepper.   Grill the sweet potatoes for 15 minutes. Tips: Grill for a few more minutes if you want your sweet potatoes crispier.

82. Wood Pellet Smoked Vegetables

Servings: 6   Cooking Time: 15 Minutes
Ingredients:
- 1 ear corn, fresh, husks and silk strands removed
- 1yellow squash, sliced
- 1 red onion, cut into wedges
- 1 green pepper, cut into strips
- 1 red pepper, cut into strips
- 1 yellow pepper, cut into strips
- 1 cup mushrooms, halved
- 2 tbsp oil
- 2 tbsp chicken seasoning

Directions:
Soak the pecan wood pellets in water for an hour. Remove the pellets from water and fill the smoker box with the wet pellets.   Place the smoker box under the grill and close the lid. Heat the grill on high heat for 10 minutes or until smoke starts coming out from the wood chips.   Meanwhile, toss the veggies in oil and seasonings then transfer them into a grill basket.   Grill for 10 minutes while turning occasionally. Serve and enjoy.
Nutrition Info: Calories 97, Total fat 5g, Saturated fat 2g, Total Carbs 11g, Net Carbs 8g, Protein 2g, Sugar 1g, Fiber 3g, Sodium: 251mg, Potassium 171mg

83. Coconut Bacon

Servings: 2   Cooking Time: 30 Minutes
Ingredients:
- 3 1/2 cups flaked coconut
- 1 tbsp pure maple syrup
- 1 tbsp water
- 2 tbsp liquid smoke
- 1 tbsp soy sauce
- 1 tsp smoked paprika (optional)

Directions:

Preheat the smoker at 325°F. Take a large mixing bowl and combine liquid smoke, maple syrup, soy sauce, and water. Pour flaked coconut over the mixture. Add it to a cooking sheet. Place in the middle rack of the smoker. Smoke it for 30 minutes and every 7-8 minutes, keep flipping the sides. Serve and enjoy.
Nutrition Info: Calories: 1244 Cal Fat: 100 g Carbohydrates: 70 g Protein: 16 g Fiber: 2 g

84. Wood Pellet Grilled Mexican Street Corn

Servings: 6   Cooking Time: 25 Minutes
Ingredients:
- 6 ears of corn on the cob, shucked
- 1 tbsp olive oil
- Kosher salt and pepper to taste
- 1/4 cup mayo
- 1/4 cup sour cream
- 1 tbsp garlic paste
- 1/2 tbsp chili powder
- Pinch of ground red pepper
- 1/2 cup cotija cheese, crumbled
- 1/4 cup cilantro, chopped
- 6 lime wedges

Directions:
Brush the corn with oil and sprinkle with salt. Place the corn on a wood pellet grill set at 350°F. Cook for 25 minutes as you turn it occasionally. Meanwhile mix mayo, cream, garlic, chili, and red pepper until well combined. When the corn is cooked remove from the grill, let it rest for some minutes then brush with the mayo mixture. Sprinkle cotija cheese, more chili powder, and cilantro. Serve with lime wedges. Enjoy.
Nutrition Info: Calories 144, Total fat 5g, Saturated fat 2g, Total Carbs 10g, Net Carbs 10g, Protein 0g, Sugar 0g, Fiber 0g, Sodium: 136mg, Potassium 173mg

85. Garlic And Rosemary Potato Wedges

Servings: 4   Cooking Time: 1 Hour 30 Minutes
Ingredients:
- 4-6 large russet potatoes, cut into wedges
- ¼ cup olive oil
- 2garlic cloves, minced
- 2tablespoons rosemary leaves, chopped
- 2teaspoon salt
- 1teaspoon fresh ground black pepper
- 1teaspoon sugar
- 1teaspoon onion powder

Directions:
Preheat your smoker to 250 degrees Fahrenheit using maple wood   Take a large bowl and add potatoes and olive oil   Toss well   Take another small bowl and stir garlic, salt, rosemary, pepper, sugar, onion powder   Sprinkle the mix on all sides of the potato wedge   Transfer the seasoned wedge to your smoker rack and smoke for 1 and a ½ hours   Serve and enjoy!
Nutrition Info: Calories: 291 Fats: 10g Carbs: 46g Fiber: 2g

86. Roasted Peach Salsa

Servings: 6   Cooking Time: 10 Minutes
Ingredients:
- 6 whole peaches, pitted and halved
- 3 tomatoes, chopped
- 2 whole onions, chopped
- ½ cup cilantro, chopped
- 2 cloves garlic, minced
- 5 teaspoons apple cider vinegar
- ½ teaspoon salt
- ¼ teaspoon black pepper
- 2 tablespoons olive oil

Directions:
Fire the   Grill to 300F. Use desired   wood pellets when cooking. Close the lid and preheat for 15 minutes. Place the peaches on the grill grate and cook for 5 minutes on each side. Remove from the grill and allow to rest for 5 minutes. Place the peaches, tomatoes, onion, and cilantro in a salad bowl. On a smaller bowl, stir in the garlic, apple cider vinegar, salt, pepper, and olive oil. Stir until well-combined. Pour into the salad and toss to coat.
Nutrition Info: Calories per serving: 155 ;
Protein: 3.1g; Carbs: 27.6 g; Fat: 5.1g Sugar: 20g

87. Grilled Asparagus & Honey-glazed Carrots

Servings: 4   Cooking Time: 35 Minutes
Ingredients:
- 1 bunch asparagus, woody ends removed
- 2 tbsp olive oil
- 1 lb peeled carrots
- 2 tbsp honey
- Sea salt to taste
- Lemon zest to taste

Directions:
Rinse the vegetables under cold water. Splash the asparagus with oil and generously with a splash of salt. Drizzle carrots generously with honey and splash lightly with salt. Preheat your   to 350F with the lid closed for about 15 minutes. Place the carrots first on the grill and cook for about 10-15 minutes. Now place asparagus on the grill and cook both for about 15-20 minutes or until done to your liking. Top with lemon zest and enjoy.
Nutrition Info: Calories 184, Total fat 7.3g, Saturated fat 1.1g, Total carbs 28.6g, Net carbs 21g, Protein 6g, Sugars 18.5g, Fiber 7.6g, Sodium 142mg, Potassium 826mg

88. Whole Roasted Cauliflower With Garlic Parmesan Butter

Servings: 5   Cooking Time: 45 Minutes
Ingredients:
- 1/4 cup olive oil
- Salt and pepper to taste
- 1 cauliflower, fresh

- 1/2 cup butter, melted
- 1/4 cup parmesan cheese, grated
- 2 garlic cloves, minced
- 1/2 tbsp parsley, chopped

Directions:
Preheat the wood pellet grill with the lid closed for 15 minutes.   Meanwhile, brush the cauliflower with oil then season with salt and pepper.   Place the cauliflower in a cast iron and place it on a grill grate. Cook for 45 minutes or until the cauliflower is golden brown and tender.   Meanwhile, mix butter, cheese, garlic, and parsley in a mixing bowl.   In the last 20 minutes of cooking, add the butter mixture.   Remove the cauliflower from the grill and top with more cheese and parsley if you desire. Enjoy.

Nutrition Info: Calories 156, Total fat 11.1g, Saturated fat 3.4g, Total Carbs 8.8g, Net Carbs 5.1g, Protein 8.2g, Sugar 0g, Fiber 3.7g, Sodium: 316mg, Potassium 468.2mg

89. Wood Pellet Smoked Acorn Squash

Servings: 6   Cooking Time: 2 Hours
Ingredients:
- 3 tbsp olive oil
- 3 acorn squash, halved and seeded
- 1/4 cup unsalted butter
- 1/4 cup brown sugar
- 1 tbsp cinnamon, ground
- 1 tbsp chili powder
- 1 tbsp nutmeg, ground

Directions:
Brush olive oil on the acorn squash cut sides then cover the halves with foil. Poke holes on the foil to allow steam and smoke through.   Fire up the wood pellet to 225°F and smoke the squash for 1-1/2-2 hours.   Remove the squash from the smoker and allow it to sit.   Meanwhile, melt butter, sugar and spices in a saucepan. Stir well to combine.   Remove the foil from the squash and spoon the butter mixture in each squash half. Enjoy.

Nutrition Info: Calories 149, Total fat 10g, Saturated fat 5g, Total Carbs 14g, Net Carbs 12g, Protein 2g, Sugar 0g, Fiber 2g, Sodium: 19mg, Potassium 0mg

90. Smoked 3-bean Salad

Servings: 6   Cooking Time: 20 Minutes
Ingredients:
- 1 can Great Northern Beans, rinsed and drained
- 1 can Red Kidney Beans, rinsed and drained
- 1pound fresh green beans, trimmed
- 2 tablespoons olive oil
- Salt and pepper to taste
- 1 shallot, sliced thinly
- 2 tablespoons red wine vinegar
- 1 teaspoon Dijon mustard

Directions:
Fire the   Grill to 500F. Use desired wood pellets when cooking. Close the lid and preheat for 15 minutes. Place the beans in a sheet tray and drizzle with olive oil.

Season with salt and pepper to taste.   Place in the grill and cook for 20 minutes. Make sure to shake the tray for even cooking.   Once cooked, remove the beans and place in a bowl. Allow to cool first.   Add the shallots and the rest of the ingredients. Season with more salt and pepper if desired. Toss to coat the beans with the seasoning.

Nutrition Info: Calories per serving: 179; Protein: 8.2 g; Carbs: 23.5g; Fat: 6.5g Sugar: 2.2g

91. Grilled Zucchini Squash

Servings: 6   Cooking Time: 10 Minutes
Ingredients:
- 3 medium zucchinis, sliced into ¼ inch thick lengthwise
- 2 tablespoons olive oil
- 1 tablespoon sherry vinegar
- 2 thyme leaves, pulled
- Salt and pepper to taste

Directions:
Fire the   Grill to 350F. Use desired wood pellets when cooking. Close the lid and preheat for 15 minutes. Place zucchini in a bowl and all ingredients. Gently massage the zucchini slices to coat with the seasoning. Place the zucchini on the grill grate and cook for 5 minutes on each side.

Nutrition Info: Calories per serving: 44; Protein: 0.3 g; Carbs: 0.9 g; Fat: 4g Sugar: 0.1g

92. Roasted Green Beans With Bacon

Servings: 6   Cooking Time: 20 Minutes
Ingredients:
- 1-pound green beans
- 4 strips bacon, cut into small pieces
- 4 tablespoons extra virgin olive oil
- 2 cloves garlic, minced
- 1 teaspoon salt

Directions:
Fire the   Grill to 400F. Use desired wood pellets when cooking. Close the lid and preheat for 15 minutes. Toss all ingredients on a sheet tray and spread out evenly. Place the tray on the grill grate and roast for 20 minutes.

Nutrition Info: Calories per serving: 65 ;
Protein: 1.3g; Carbs: 3.8g; Fat: 5.3g Sugar: 0.6g

93. Smoked Deviled Eggs

Servings: 4 To 6   Cooking Time: 50 Minutes
Ingredients:
- 6 large eggs
- 1slice bacon
- 1/4 cup mayonnaise
- 1tsp Dijon mustard
- 1tsp apple cider vinegar
- 1/4 tsp paprika
- Pinch of kosher salt
- 1tbsp chives, chopped

Directions:
Preheat pellet grill to 180°F and turn smoke setting on, if applicable.   Bring a pot of water to a boil. Add eggs and hard boil eggs for about 12 minutes.   Remove eggs from pot and place them into an ice-water bath. Once eggs have cooled completely, peel them and slice in half lengthwise.   Place sliced eggs on grill, yolk side up. Smoke for 30 to 45 minutes, depending on how much smoky flavor you want.   While eggs smoke, cook bacon until it's crispy.   Remove eggs from the grill and allow to cool on a plate.   Remove the yolks and place all of them in a small bowl. Place the egg whites on a plate.   Mash yolks with a fork and add mayonnaise, mustard, apple cider vinegar, paprika, and salt. Stir until combined.   Spoon a scoop of yolk mixture back into each egg white.   Sprinkle paprika, chives, and crispy bacon bits to garnish. Serve and enjoy!
Nutrition Info: Calories: 140 Fat: 12 g Cholesterol: 190 mg Carbohydrate: 1 g Fiber: 0 Sugar: 0 Protein: 6 g

94. Twice-smoked Potatoes

Servings: 16   Cooking Time: 1 Hour 35 Minutes
Ingredients:
- 8 Idaho, Russet, or Yukon Gold potatoes
- 1 (12-ounce) can evaporated milk, heated
- 1 cup (2 sticks) butter, melted
- ½ cup sour cream, at room temperature
- 1 cup grated Parmesan cheese
- ½ pound bacon, cooked and crumbled
- ¼ cup chopped scallions
- Salt
- Freshly ground black pepper
- 1 cup shredded Cheddar cheese

Directions:
Supply your smoker with wood pellets and follow the manufacturer's specific start-up procedure. Preheat, with the lid closed, to 400°F.   Poke the potatoes all over with a fork. Arrange them directly on the grill grate, close the lid, and smoke for 1 hour and 15 minutes, or until cooked through and they have some give when pinched.   Let the potatoes cool for 10 minutes, then cut in half lengthwise.   Into a medium bowl, scoop out the potato flesh, leaving ¼ inch in the shells; place the shells on a baking sheet.   Using an electric mixer on medium speed, beat the potatoes, milk, butter, and sour cream until smooth.   Stir in the Parmesan cheese, bacon, and scallions, and season with salt and pepper. Generously stuff each shell with the potato mixture and top with Cheddar cheese.   Place the baking sheet on the grill grate, close the lid, and smoke for 20 minutes, or until the cheese is melted.

95. Wood Pellet Grilled Zucchini Squash Spears

Servings: 5   Cooking Time: 10 Minutes
Ingredients:
- 4 zucchini, cleaned and ends cut
- 2 tbsp olive oil

- 1 tbsp sherry vinegar
- 2 thyme, leaves pulled
- Salt and pepper to taste

Directions:
Cut the zucchini into halves then cut each half thirds. Add the rest of the ingredients in a ziplock bag with the zucchini pieces. Toss to mix well.   Preheat the wood pellet temperature to 350°F with the lid closed for 15 minutes.   Remove the zucchini from the bag and place them on the grill grate with the cut side down.   Cook for 4 minutes per side or until the zucchini are tender. Remove from grill and serve with thyme leaves. Enjoy.
Nutrition Info: Calories 74, Total fat 5.4g, Saturated fat 0.5g, Total Carbs 6.1g, Net Carbs 3.8g, Protein 2.6g, Sugar 3.9g, Fiber 2.3g, Sodium: 302mg, Potassium 599mg

96. Mexican Street Corn With Chipotle Butter 2

Servings: 6   Cooking Time: 45 Minutes
Ingredients:
- 16 to 20 long toothpicks
- 1 pound Brussels sprouts, trimmed and wilted, leaves removed
- ½ pound bacon, cut in half
- 1 tablespoon packed brown sugar
- 1 tablespoon Cajun seasoning
- ¼ cup balsamic vinegar
- ¼ cup extra-virgin olive oil
- ¼ cup chopped fresh cilantro
- 2 teaspoons minced garlic

Directions:
Soak the toothpicks in water for 15 minutes.   Supply your smoker with wood pellets and follow the manufacturer's specific start-up procedure. Preheat, with the lid closed, to 300°F.   Wrap each Brussels sprout in a half slice of bacon and secure with a toothpick. In a small bowl, combine the brown sugar and Cajun seasoning. Dip each wrapped Brussels sprout in this sweet rub and roll around to coat.   Place the sprouts on a Frogmat or parchment paper–lined baking sheet on the grill grate, close the lid, and smoke for 45 minutes to 1 hour, turning as needed, until cooked evenly and the bacon is crisp.   In a small bowl, whisk together the balsamic vinegar, olive oil, cilantro, and garlic. Remove the toothpicks from the Brussels sprouts, transfer to a plate and serve drizzled with the cilantro-balsamic sauce.

97. Wood Pellet Grill Spicy Sweet Potatoes

Servings: 6   Cooking Time: 35 Minutes
Ingredients:
- 2 lb sweet potatoes, cut into chunks
- 1 red onion, chopped
- 2 tbsp oil
- 2 tbsp orange juice
- 1 tbsp roasted cinnamon
- 1 tbsp salt

- 1/4 tbsp Chiptole chili pepper

Directions:
Preheat the wood pellet grill to 425°F with the lid closed. Toss the sweet potatoes with onion, oil, and juice. In a mixing bowl, mix cinnamon, salt, and pepper then sprinkle the mixture over the sweet potatoes. Spread the potatoes on a lined baking dish in a single layer. Place the baking dish in the grill and grill for 30 minutes or until the sweet potatoes ate tender. Serve and enjoy.

Nutrition Info: Calories 145, Total fat 5g, Saturated fat 0g, Total Carbs 23g, Net Carbs 19g, Protein 2g, Sugar 3g, Fiber 4g, Sodium: 428mg, Potassium 230mg

98. Roasted Root Vegetables

Servings: 6   Cooking Time: 45 Minutes
Ingredients:
- 1 large red onion, peeled
- 1 bunch of red beets, trimmed, peeled
- 1 large yam, peeled
- 1 bunch of golden beets, trimmed, peeled
- 1 large parsnips, peeled
- 1 butternut squash, peeled
- 1 large carrot, peeled
- 6 garlic cloves, peeled
- 3 tablespoons thyme leaves
- Salt as needed
- 1 cinnamon stick
- Ground black pepper as needed
- 3 tablespoons olive oil
- 2 tablespoons honey

Directions:
Switch on the grill, fill the grill hopper with hickory flavored wood pellets, power the grill on by using the control panel, select 'smoke' on the temperature dial, or set the temperature to 450 degrees F and let it preheat for a minimum of 15 minutes. Meanwhile, cut all the vegetables into ½-inch pieces, place them in a large bowl, add garlic, thyme, and cinnamon, drizzle with oil and toss until mixed. Take a large cookie sheet, line it with foil, spread with vegetables, and then season with salt and black pepper. When the grill has preheated, open the lid, place prepared cookie sheet on the grill grate, shut the grill and smoke for 45 minutes until tender. When done, transfer vegetables to a dish, drizzle with honey, and then serve.

Nutrition Info: Calories: 164 Cal ;Fat: 4 g ;Carbs: 31.7 g ;Protein: 2.7 g ;Fiber: 6.4 g

99. Split Pea Soup With Mushrooms

Servings: 4   Cooking Time: 35 Minutes
Ingredients:
- 2tbsp. Olive Oil
- 3Garlic cloves, minced
- 3tbsp. Parsley, fresh and chopped
- 2Carrots chopped
- 1.2/3 cup Green Peas
- 9cups Water
- 2tsp. Salt
- 1/4 tsp. Black Pepper
- 1lb. Portobello Mushrooms
- 1Bay Leaf
- 2Celery Ribs, chopped
- 1Onion quartered
- 1/2 tsp. Thyme, dried
- 6tbsp. Parmesan Cheese, grated

Directions:
First, keep oil, onion, and garlic in the blender pitcher. Next, select the 'saute' button. Once sautéed, stir in the rest of the ingredients, excluding parsley and cheese. Then, press the 'hearty soup' button. Finally, transfer the soup among the serving bowls and garnish it with parsley and cheese.

Nutrition Info: Calories: 61 Fat: 1.1 g Total Carbs: 10 g Fiber: 1.9 g Sugar: 3.2 g Protein: 3.2 g Cholesterol: 0

100. Smoked Cherry Tomatoes

Servings: 8-10   Cooking Time: 1 ½ Hours
Ingredients:
- 2 pints of tomatoes

Directions:
Preheat the electric smoker to 225°F while adding wood chips and water to the smoker. Clean the tomatoes with clean water and dry them off properly. Place the tomatoes on the pan and place the pan in the smoker. Smoke for 90 minutes while adding water and wood chips to the smoker.

Nutrition Info: Calories: 16 Cal Fat: 0 g Carbohydrates: 3 g   Protein: 1 g Fiber: 1 g

FISH AND SEAFOOD RECIPES

101. Juicy Smoked Salmon

Servings: 5   Cooking Time: 50 Minutes
Ingredients:
- ½ cup of sugar
- 2 tablespoon salt
- 2 tablespoons crushed red pepper flakes
- ½ cup fresh mint leaves, chopped
- ¼ cup brandy
- 1(4 pounds) salmon, bones removed
- 2cups alder wood pellets, soaked in water

Directions:
Take a medium-sized bowl and add brown sugar, crushed red pepper flakes, mint leaves, salt, and brandy until a paste forms   Rub the paste all over your salmon and wrap the salmon with a plastic wrap   Allow them to chill overnight   Preheat your smoker to 220 degrees Fahrenheit and add wood Pellets   Transfer the salmon to the smoker rack and cook smoke for 45 minutes   Once the salmon has turned red-brown and the flesh flakes off easily, take it out and serve!
Nutrition Info: Calories: 370 Fats: 28g Carbs: 1g Fiber: 0g

102. Wood Pellet Grilled Scallops

Servings: 4   Cooking Time: 15 Minutes
Ingredients:
- 2 lb sea scallops, dried with a paper towel
- 1/2 tbsp garlic salt
- 2 tbsp kosher salt
- 4 tbsp salted butter
- Squeeze lemon juice

Directions:
Preheat the wood pellet grill to 400°F with the cast pan inside.   Sprinkle with both salts, pepper on both sides of the scallops.   Place the butter on the cast iron then add the scallops. Close the lid and cook for 8 minutes. Flip the scallops and close the lid once more. Cook for 8 more minutes.   Remove the scallops from the grill and give a lemon squeeze. Serve immediately and enjoy.
Nutrition Info: Calories 177, Total fat 7g, Saturated fat 4g, Total Carbs 6g, Net Carbs 6g, Protein 23g, Sugar 0g, Fiber 0g, Sodium: 1430mg, Potassium 359mg

103. Lemon Garlic Scallops

Servings: 6   Cooking Time: 5 Minutes
Ingredients:
- 1 dozen scallops
- 2 tablespoons chopped parsley
- Salt as needed
- 1 tablespoon olive oil
- 1 tablespoon butter, unsalted
- 1 teaspoon lemon zest
- For the Garlic Butter:
- ½ teaspoon minced garlic
- 1 lemon, juiced
- 4 tablespoons butter, unsalted, melted

Directions:
Switch on the   grill, fill the grill hopper with alder flavored wood pellets, power the grill on by using the control panel, select 'smoke' on the temperature dial, or set the temperature to 400 degrees F and let it preheat for a minimum of 15 minutes.   Meanwhile, remove frill from scallops, pat dry with paper towels and then season with salt and black pepper.   When the grill has preheated, open the lid, place a skillet on the grill grate, add butter and oil, and when the butter melts, place seasoned scallops on it and then cook for 2 minutes until seared.   Meanwhile, prepare the garlic butter and for this, take a small bowl, place all of its ingredients in it and then whisk until combined.   Flip the scallops, top with some of the prepared garlic butter, and cook for another minute.   When done, transfer scallops to a dish, top with remaining garlic butter, sprinkle with parsley and lemon zest, and then serve.
Nutrition Info: Calories: 184 Cal ;Fat: 10 g ;Carbs: 1 g ;Protein: 22 g ;Fiber: 0.2 g

104. Yummy Buttery Clams

Servings: 6   Cooking Time: 8 Minutes
Ingredients:
- 24 littleneck clams
- ½ C. cold butter, chopped
- 2 tbsp. fresh parsley, minced
- 3 garlic cloves, minced
- 1 tsp. fresh lemon juice

Directions:
Set the temperature of   Grill to 450 degrees F and preheat with closed lid for 15 minutes.   Scrub the clams under cold running water.   In a large casserole dish, mix together remaining ingredients.   Place the casserole dish onto the grill.   Now, arrange the clams directly onto the grill and cook for about 5-8 minutes or until they are opened. (Discard any that fail to open). With tongs, carefully transfer the opened clams into the casserole dish and remove from grill.   Serve immediately.
Nutrition Info: Calories per serving: 306; Carbohydrates: 6.4g; Protein: 29.3g; Fat: 7.6g; Sugar: 0.1g; Sodium: 237mg; Fiber: 0.1g

105. Rockfish

Servings: 6   Cooking Time: 20 Minutes
Ingredients:
- 6 rockfish fillets
- 1 lemon, sliced
- 3/4 tbsp salt
- 2 tbsp fresh dill, chopped
- 1/2 tbsp garlic powder

- 1/2 tbsp onion powder
- 6 tbsp butter

Directions:
Preheat your to 400F. Season the fish with salt, dill, garlic and onion powder on both sides then place it in a baking dish. Place a pat of butter and a lemon slice on each fillet. Place the baking dish in the and close the lid. Cook for 20 minutes or until the fish is no longer translucent and is flaky. Remove from and let rest for 5 minutes before serving.

Nutrition Info: Calories 270, Total fat 17g, Saturated fat 9g, Total carbs 2g, Net carbs 2g Protein 28g, Sugars 0g, Fiber 0g, Sodium 381mg

106. Super-tasty Trout

Servings: 8   Cooking Time: 5 Hours
Ingredients:
- 1 (7-lb.) whole lake trout, butterflied
- ½ C. kosher salt
- ½ C. fresh rosemary, chopped
- 2 tsp. lemon zest, grated finely

Directions:
Rub the trout with salt generously and then, sprinkle with rosemary and lemon zest. Arrange the trout in a large baking dish and refrigerate for about 7-8 hours. Remove the trout from baking dish and rinse under cold running water to remove the salt. With paper towels, pat dry the trout completely. Arrange a wire rack in a sheet pan. Place the trout onto the wire rack, skin side down and refrigerate for about 24 hours. Set the temperature of Grill to 180 degrees F and preheat with closed lid for 15 minutes, using charcoal. Place the trout onto the grill and cook for about 2-4 hours or until desired doneness. Remove the trout from grill and place onto a cutting board for about 5 minutes before serving.

Nutrition Info: Calories per serving: 633; Carbohydrates: 2.4g; Protein: 85.2g; Fat: 31.8g; Sugar: 0g; Sodium: 5000mg; Fiber: 1.6g

107. Salmon With Togarashi

Servings: 3   Cooking Time: 20 Minutes
Ingredients:
- 1 salmon fillet
- 1/4 cup olive oil
- 1/2 tbsp kosher salt
- 1 tbsp Togarashi seasoning

Directions:
Preheat your to 400F. Place the salmon on a sheet lined with non-stick foil with the skin side down. Rub the oil into the meat then sprinkle salt and Togarashi. Place the salmon on the grill and cook for 20 minutes or until the internal temperature reaches 145F with the lid closed. Remove from the and serve when hot.

Nutrition Info: Calories 119, Total fat 10g, Saturated fat 2g, Total carbs 0g, Net carbs 0g Protein 0g, Sugars 0g, Fiber 0g, Sodium 720mg

108. Grilled Herbed Tuna

Servings: 6   Cooking Time: 10 Minutes
Ingredients:
- 6 tuna steaks
- 1 tablespoon lemon zest
- 1 tablespoon fresh thyme, chopped
- 1 tablespoon fresh parsley, chopped
- Garlic salt to taste

Directions:
Sprinkle the tuna steaks with lemon zest, herbs and garlic salt. Cover with foil. Refrigerate for 4 hours. Grill for 3 minutes per side. Tips: Take the fish out of the refrigerator 30 minutes before cooking.

109. Peppercorn Tuna Steaks

Servings: 3   Cooking Time: 10 Minutes
Ingredients:
- ¼ cup of salt
- 2 pounds yellowfin tuna
- ¼ cup Dijon mustard
- Freshly ground black pepper
- 2 tablespoons peppercorn

Directions:
Take a large-sized container and dissolve salt in warm water (enough water to cover fish) Transfer tuna to the brine and cover, refrigerate for 8 hours Preheat your smoker to 250 degrees Fahrenheit with your preferred wood Remove tuna from bring and pat it dry Transfer to grill pan and spread Dijon mustard all over Season with pepper and sprinkle peppercorn on top Transfer tuna to smoker and smoker for 1 hour Enjoy!

Nutrition Info: Calories: 707 Fats: 57g Carbs: 10g Fiber: 2g

110. Grilled Tilapia

Servings: 6   Cooking Time: 2o Minutes
Ingredients:
- 2 tsp dried parsley
- ½ tsp garlic powder
- 1 tsp cayenne pepper
- ½ tsp ground black pepper
- ½ tsp thyme
- ½ tsp dried basil
- ½ tsp oregano
- 3 tbsp olive oil
- ½ tsp lemon pepper
- 1 tsp kosher salt
- 1 lemon (juiced)
- 6 tilapia fillets
- 1 ½ tsp creole seafood seasoning

Directions:
In a mixing bowl, combine spices Brush the fillets with oil and lemon juice. Liberally, season all sides of the tilapia fillets with the seasoning mix. Preheat your grill to 325°F Place a non-stick BBQ grilling try on the

grill and arrange the tilapia fillets onto it.   Grill for 15 to 20 minutes   Remove fillets and cool down
Nutrition Info: Calories: 176 Cal Fat: 9.6 g Carbohydrates: 1.5 g   Protein: 22.3 g Fiber: 0.5 g

111. Cajun Seasoned Shrimp

Servings: 4   Cooking Time: 16-20 Minutes
Ingredients:
- 20 pieces of jumbo Shrimp
- 1/2 teaspoon of Cajun seasoning
- 1tablespoon of Canola oil
- 1teaspoon of magic shrimp seasoning

Directions:
Take a large bowl and add canola oil, shrimp, and seasonings.   Mix well for fine coating.   Now put the shrimp on skewers.   Put the grill grate inside the grill and set a timer to 8 minutes at high for preheating. Once the grill is preheated, open the unit and place the shrimp skewers inside.   Cook the shrimp for 2 minutes. Open the unit to flip the shrimp and cook for another 2 minutes at medium.   Own done, serve.
Nutrition Info: Calories: 382 Total Fat: 7.4g Saturated Fat: 0g Cholesterol: 350mg Sodium: 2208mg Total Carbohydrate: 23.9g Dietary Fiber 2.6g Total Sugars: 2.6g Protein: 50.2g

112. Wood Pellet Teriyaki Smoked Shrimp

Servings: 6   Cooking Time: 10 Minutes
Ingredients:
- 1 lb tail-on shrimp, uncooked
- 1/2 tbsp onion powder
- 1/2 tbsp salt
- 1/2 tbsp Garlic powder
- 4 tbsp Teriyaki sauce
- 4 tbsp sriracha mayo
- 2 tbsp green onion, minced

Directions:
Peel the shrimps leaving the tails then wash them removing any vein left over. Drain and pat with a paper towel to drain.   Preheat the wood pellet to 450°F Season the shrimp with onion, salt, and garlic then place it on the grill to cook for 5 minutes on each side. Remove the shrimp from the grill and toss it with teriyaki sauce. Serve garnished with mayo and onions. Enjoy.
Nutrition Info: Calories 87, Total fat 0g, Saturated fat 0g, Total Carbs 2g, Net Carbs 2g, Protein 16g, Sugar 1g, Fiber 0g, Sodium: 1241mg

113. Bacon-wrapped Scallops

Servings: 4   Cooking Time: 30 Minutes
Ingredients:
- 12 scallops
- 12 bacon slices
- 3 tablespoons lemon juice
- Pepper to taste

Directions:

Turn on your wood pellet grill.   Set it to smoke.   Let it burn for 5 minutes while the lid is open.   Set it to 400 degrees F.   Wrap the scallops with bacon.   Secure with a toothpick.   Drizzle with the lemon juice and season with pepper.   Add the scallops to a baking tray. Place the tray on the grill.   Grill for 20 minutes. Serving Suggestion: Serve with sweet chili sauce.
Nutrition Info: Calories: 180.3 Fat: 8 g Cholesterol: 590.2 mg Carbohydrates: 3 g Fiber: 0 g Sugars: 0 g Protein: 22 g

114. Bacon-wrapped Scallops

Servings: 8   Cooking Time: 20 Minutes
Ingredients:
- 1 lb sea scallops
- 1/2 lb bacon
- Sea salt

Directions:
Preheat your   to 375F.   Pat dry the scallops with a paper towel then wrap them with a piece of bacon and secure with a toothpick.   Lay the scallops on the grill with the bacon side down. Close the lid and cook for 5 minutes on each side.   Keep the scallops on the bacon side so that you will not get grill marks on the scallops. Serve and enjoy.
Nutrition Info: Calories 261, Total fat 14g, Saturated fat 5g, Total carbs 5g, Net carbs 5g Protein 28g, Sugars 0g, Fiber 0g, Sodium 1238mg

115. Barbecued Shrimp

Servings: 4   Cooking Time: 10 Minutes
Ingredients:
- 1 pound peeled and deveined shrimp, with tails on
- 2 tablespoons olive oil
- 1 batch Dill Seafood Rub

Directions:
Soak wooden skewers in water for 30 minutes.   Supply your smoker with wood pellets and follow the manufacturer's specific start-up procedure. Preheat the grill, with the lid closed, to 375°F.   Thread 4 or 5 shrimp per skewer.   Coat the shrimp all over with olive oil and season each side of the skewers with the rub. Place the skewers directly on the grill grate and grill the shrimp for 5 minutes per side. Remove the skewers from the grill and serve immediately.

116. Oyster In Shells

Servings: 4   Cooking Time: 8 Minutes
Ingredients:
- 12 medium oysters
- 1 tsp oregano
- 1 lemon (juiced)
- 1 tsp freshly ground black pepper
- 6 tbsp unsalted butter (melted)
- 1 tsp salt or more to taste
- 2 garlic cloves (minced)

- 2 ½ tbsp grated parmesan cheese
- 2 tbsp freshly chopped parsley

Directions:
Remove dirt   Open the shell completely. Discard the top shell.   Gently run the knife under the oyster to loosen the oyster foot from the bottom shell.   Repeat step 2 and 3 for the remaining oysters.   Combine melted butter, lemon, pepper, salt, garlic and oregano in a mixing bowl.   Pour ½ to 1 tsp of the butter mixture on each oyster.   Start your wood pellet grill on smoke, leaving the lid opened for 5 minutes, or until fire starts. Keep lid unopened to preheat in the set "HIGH" with lid closed for 15 minutes.   Gently arrange the oysters onto the grill grate.   Grill oyster for 6 to 8 minutes or until the oyster juice is bubbling and the oyster is plump. Remove oysters from heat. Serve and top with grated parmesan and chopped parsley.

Nutrition Info: Calories: 200 Cal Fat: 19.2 g Carbohydrates: 3.9 g   Protein: 4.6 g Fiber: 0.8 g

117. Grilled King Crab Legs

Servings: 4   Cooking Time: 25 Minutes
Ingredients:
- 4 pounds king crab legs (split)
- 4 tbsp lemon juice
- 2 tbsp garlic powder
- 1 cup butter (melted)
- 2 tsp brown sugar
- 2 tsp paprika
- Black pepper (depends to your liking)

Directions:
In a mixing bowl, combine the lemon juice, butter, sugar, garlic, paprika and pepper.   Arrange the split crab on a baking sheet, split side up. Drizzle ¾ of the butter mixture over the crab legs. Configure your pellet grill for indirect cooking and preheat it to 225°F, using mesquite wood pellets.   Arrange the crab legs onto the grill grate, shell side down. Cover the grill and cook 25 minutes. Remove the crab legs from the grill. Serve and top with the remaining butter mixture.

Nutrition Info: Calories: 480 Cal Fat: 53.2 g Carbohydrates: 6.1 g   Protein: 88.6 g Fiber: 1.2 g

118. Crazy Delicious Lobster Tails

Servings: 4   Cooking Time: 25 Minutes
Ingredients:
- ½ C. butter, melted
- 2 garlic cloves, minced
- 2 tsp. fresh lemon juice
- Salt and freshly ground black pepper, to taste
- 4 (8-oz.) lobster tails

Directions:
Set the temperature of   Grill to 450 degrees F and preheat with closed lid for 15 minutes.   In a metal pan, add all ingredients except for lobster tails and mix well. Place the pan onto the grill and cook for about 10 minutes.   Meanwhile, cut down the top of the shell and expose lobster meat.   Remove pan of butter mixture from grill.   Coat the lobster meat with butter mixture. Place the lobster tails onto the grill and cook for about 15 minutes, coating with butter mixture once halfway through.   Remove from grill and serve hot.

Nutrition Info: Calories per serving: 409; Carbohydrates: 0.6g; Protein: 43.5g; Fat: 24.9g; Sugar: 0.1g; Sodium: 1305mg; Fiber: 0g

119. Seared Tuna Steaks

Servings: 2   Cooking Time: 10 Minutes
Ingredients:
- 2 (1½- to 2-inch-thick) tuna steaks
- 2 tablespoons olive oil
- Salt
- Freshly ground black pepper

Directions:
Supply your smoker with wood pellets and follow the manufacturer's specific start-up procedure. Preheat the grill, with the lid closed, to 500°F.   Rub the tuna steaks all over with olive oil and season both sides with salt and pepper.   Place the tuna steaks directly on the grill grate and grill for 3 to 5 minutes per side, leaving a pink center. Remove the tuna steaks from the grill and serve immediately.

120. Jerk Shrimp

Servings: 12   Cooking Time: 6 Minutes
Ingredients:
- 2 pounds shrimp, peeled, deveined
- 3 tablespoons olive oil
- For the Spice Mix:
- 1 teaspoon garlic powder
- 1 teaspoon of sea salt
- 1/4 teaspoon ground cayenne
- 1 tablespoon brown sugar
- 1/8 teaspoon smoked paprika
- 1 tablespoon smoked paprika
- 1/4 teaspoon ground thyme
- 1 lime, zested

Directions:
Switch on the   grill, fill the grill hopper with flavored wood pellets, power the grill on by using the control panel, select 'smoke' on the temperature dial, or set the temperature to 450 degrees F and let it preheat for a minimum of 5 minutes.   Meanwhile, prepare the spice mix and for this, take a small bowl, place all of its ingredients in it and stir until mixed.   Take a large bowl, place shrimps in it, sprinkle with prepared spice mix, drizzle with oil and toss until well coated.   When the grill has preheated, open the lid, place shrimps on the grill grate, shut the grill and smoke for 3 minutes per side until firm and thoroughly cooked.   When done, transfer shrimps to a dish and then serve.

Nutrition Info: Calories: 131 Cal ;Fat: 4.3 g ;Carbs: 0 g ;Protein: 22 g ;Fiber: 0 g

121. Bacon-wrapped Shrimp

Servings: 12   Cooking Time: 10 Minutes
Ingredients:
- 1 lb raw shrimp
- 1/2 tbsp salt
- 1/4 tbsp garlic powder
- 1 lb bacon, cut into halves

Directions:
Preheat your   to 350F.   Remove the shells and tails from the shrimp then pat them dry with the paper towels. Sprinkle salt and garlic on the shrimp then wrap with bacon and secure with a toothpick.   Place the shrimps on a baking rack greased with cooking spray.   Cook for 10 minutes, flip and cook for another 10 minutes or until the bacon is crisp enough.   Remove from the   and serve.

Nutrition Info: Calories 204, Total fat 14g, Saturated fat 5g, Total carbs 1g, Net carbs 1g Protein 18g, Sugars 0g, Fiber 0g, Sodium 939mg

122. Lobster Tail

Servings: 2   Cooking Time: 25 Minutes
Ingredients:
- 2 lobster tails
- Salt
- Freshly ground black pepper
- 1 batch Lemon Butter Mop for Seafood

Directions:
Supply your smoker with wood pellets and follow the manufacturer's specific start-up procedure. Preheat the grill, with the lid closed, to 375°F.   Using kitchen shears, slit the top of the lobster shells, through the center, nearly to the tail. Once cut, expose as much meat as you can through the cut shell.   Season the lobster tails all over with salt and pepper.   Place the tails directly on the grill grate and grill until their internal temperature reaches 145°F. Remove the lobster from the grill and serve with the mop on the side for dipping.

123. Grilled Salmon

Servings: 4   Cooking Time: 25 Minutes
Ingredients:
- 1 (2-pound) half salmon fillet
- 3 tablespoons mayonnaise
- 1 batch Dill Seafood Rub

Directions:
Supply your smoker with wood pellets and follow the manufacturer's specific start-up procedure. Preheat the grill, with the lid closed, to 325°F.   Using your hands, rub the salmon fillet all over with the mayonnaise and sprinkle it with the rub.   Place the salmon directly on the grill grate, skin-side down, and grill until its internal temperature reaches 145°F. Remove the salmon from the grill and serve immediately.

124. Hot-smoked Salmon

Servings: 4   Cooking Time: 4 To 6 Hours
Ingredients:
- 1 (2-pound) half salmon fillet
- 1 batch Dill Seafood Rub

Directions:
Supply your smoker with wood pellets and follow the manufacturer's specific start-up procedure. Preheat the grill, with the lid closed, to 180°F.   Season the salmon all over with the rub. Using your hands, work the rub into the flesh.   Place the salmon directly on the grill grate, skin-side down, and smoke until its internal temperature reaches 145°F. Remove the salmon from the grill and serve immediately.

125. Spot Prawn Skewers

Servings: 6   Cooking Time: 10 Minutes
Ingredients:
- 2 lb spot prawns
- 2 tbsp oil
- Salt and pepper to taste

Directions:
Preheat your   to 400F.   Skewer your prawns with soaked skewers then generously sprinkle with oil, salt, and pepper.   Place the skewers on the grill and cook with the lid closed for 5 minutes on each side.   Remove the skewers and serve when hot.

Nutrition Info: Calories 221, Total fat 7g, Saturated fat 1g, Total carbs 2g, Net carbs 2g Protein 34g, Sugars 0g, Fiber 0g, Sodium 1481mg

126. Wood Pellet Grilled Salmon Sandwich

Servings: 4   Cooking Time: 15 Minutes
Ingredients:
- Salmon Sandwiches
- 4 salmon fillets
- 1 tbsp olive oil
- Fin and feather rub
- 1 tbsp salt
- 4 toasted bun
- Butter lettuce
- Dill Aioli
- 1/2 cup mayonnaise
- 1/2 tbsp lemon zest
- 2 tbsp lemon juice
- 1/4 tbsp salt
- 1/2 tbsp fresh dill, minced

Directions:
Mix all the dill aioli ingredients and place them in the fridge.   Preheat the wood pellet grill to 450°F. Brush the salmon fillets with oil, rub, and salt. Place the fillets on the grill and cook until the internal temperature reaches 135°F.   Remove the fillets from the grill and let rest for 5 minutes.   Spread the aioli on the buns then top with salmon, lettuce, and the top bun.   Serve when hot.

Nutrition Info: Calories 852, Total fat 54g, Saturated fat 10g, Total Carbs 30g, Net Carbs 28g, Protein 57g, Sugar 5g, Fiber 2g, Sodium: 1268mg, Potassium 379mg

127. Wood Pellet Togarashi Grilled Salmon

Servings: 6   Cooking Time: 20 Minutes
Ingredients:
- 1 salmon fillet
- 1/4 cup olive oil
- 1/2 tbsp kosher salt
- 1 tbsp Togarashi seasoning

Directions:
Preheat the wood pellet grill to 400°F.   Place the salmon fillet on a non-stick foil sheet with the skin side up.   Rub the olive oil on the salmon and sprinkle with salt and togarashi seasoning.   Place the salmon on the preheated grill and close the lid. Cook for 20 minutes or until the internal temperature reaches 145°F.   Remove from the grill and serve when hot. Enjoy.
Nutrition Info: Calories 119, Total fat 10g, Saturated fat 2g, Total Carbs 0g, Net Carbs 0g, Protein 6g, Sugar 0g, Fiber 0g, Sodium: 720mg

128. Chilean Sea Bass

Servings: 6   Cooking Time: 40 Minutes
Ingredients:
- 4 sea bass fillets, skinless, each about 6 ounces
- Chicken rub as needed
- 8 tablespoons butter, unsalted
- 2 tablespoons chopped thyme leaves
- Lemon slices for serving
- For the Marinade:
- 1 lemon, juiced
- 4 teaspoons minced garlic
- 1 tablespoon chopped thyme
- 1 teaspoon blackened rub
- 1 tablespoon chopped oregano
- 1/4 cup oil

Directions:
Prepare the marinade and for this, take a small bowl, place all of its ingredients in it, stir until well combined, and then pour the mixture into a large plastic bag. Add fillets in the bag, seal it, turn it upside down to coat fillets with the marinade and let it marinate for a minimum of 30 minutes in the refrigerator.   When ready to cook, switch on the   grill, fill the grill hopper with apple-flavored wood pellets, power the grill on by using the control panel, select 'smoke' on the temperature dial, or set the temperature to 325 degrees F and let it preheat for a minimum of 15 minutes. Meanwhile, take a large baking pan and place butter on it.   When the grill has preheated, open the lid, place baking pan on the grill grate, and wait until butter melts. Remove fillets from the marinade, pour marinade into the pan with melted butter, then season fillets with chicken rubs until coated on all sides, then place them into the pan, shut the grill and cook for 30 minutes until internal temperature reaches 160 degrees F, frequently

basting with the butter sauce.   When done, transfer fillets to a dish, sprinkle with thyme and then serve with lemon slices.
Nutrition Info: Calories: 232 Cal ;Fat: 12.2 g ;Carbs: 0.8 g ;Protein: 28.2 g ;Fiber: 0.1 g

129. Grilled Shrimp

Servings: 4   Cooking Time: 15 Minutes
Ingredients:
- Jumbo shrimp peeled and cleaned - 1 lb.
- Oil - 2 tbsp
- Salt - ½ tbsp
- Skewers - 4-5
- Pepper - ⅛ tbsp
- Garlic salt - ½ tbsp

Directions:
Preheat the wood pellet grill to 375 degrees.   Mix all the ingredients in a small bowl.   After washing and drying the shrimp, mix it well with the oil and seasonings. Add skewers to the shrimp and set the bowl of shrimp aside.   Open the skewers and flip them.   Cook for 4 more minutes. Remove when the shrimp is opaque and pink.
Nutrition Info: Carbohydrates: 1.3 g Protein: 19 g Fat: 1.4 g Sodium: 805 mg   Cholesterol: 179 mg

130. Mussels With Pancetta Aïoli

Servings: 4   Cooking Time: 30 Minutes
Ingredients:
- ¾ cup mayonnaise (to make your own, see page 460)
- 1tablespoon minced garlic, or more to taste
- 1.4-ounce slice pancetta, chopped
- Salt and pepper
- 4 pounds mussels
- 8 thick slices Italian bread
- ¼ cup good-quality olive oil

Directions:
Whisk the mayonnaise and garlic together in a small bowl. Put the pancetta in a small cold skillet, turn the heat to low; cook, occasionally stir, until most of the fat is rendered and the meat turns golden and crisp about 5 minutes. Drain on a paper towel, then stir into the mayonnaise along with 1 teaspoon of the rendered fat from the pan. Taste and add more garlic and some salt if you like. Cover and refrigerate until you're ready to serve. (You can make the aïoli up to several days ahead; refrigerate in an airtight container.)   Start the coals or heat a gas grill for direct hot cooking. Make sure the grates are clean.   Rinse the mussels and pull off any beards. Discard any that are broken or don't close when tapped.   Brush both sides of the bread slices with the oil. Put the bread on the grill directly over the fire. Close the lid and toast, turning once, until it develops grill marks with some charring, 1 to 2 minutes per side. Remove from the grill and keep warm.   Scatter the mussels onto the grill directly over the fire, spreading them out, so they are in a single layer. Immediately close

the lid and cook for 3 minutes. Transfer the open mussels to a large bowl with tongs. If any have not opened, leave them on the grill, close the lid, and cook for another minute or 2, checking frequently and removing open mussels until they are all off the grill.   Dollop the aïoli over the tops of the mussels and use a large spoon to turn them over to coat them. Serve the mussels drizzled with their juices, either over (or alongside) the bread.
Nutrition Info: Calories: 159 Fats: 6.1 g Cholesterol: 0 mg Carbohydrates: 14.95 g Fiber: 0 g Sugars: 0 g Proteins: 9.57 g

131. Barbeque Shrimp

Servings: 6   Cooking Time: 8 Minutes
Ingredients:
- 2-pound raw shrimp (peeled and deveined)
- ¼ cup extra virgin olive oil
- ½ tsp paprika
- ½ tsp red pepper flakes
- 2 garlic cloves (minced)
- 1 tsp cumin
- 1 lemon (juiced)
- 1 tsp kosher salt
- 1 tbsp chili paste
- Bamboo or wooden skewers (soaked for 30 minutes, at least)

Directions:
Combine the pepper flakes, cumin, lemon, salt, chili, paprika, garlic and olive oil. Add the shrimp and toss to combine.   Transfer the shrimp and marinade into a zip-lock bag and refrigerate for 4 hours.   Let shrimp rest in room temperature after pulling it out from marinade   Start your grill on smoke, leaving the lid opened for 5 minutes, or until fire starts. Use hickory wood pellet.   Keep lid unopened and preheat the grill to "high" for 15 minutes.   Thread shrimps onto skewers and arrange the skewers on the grill grate. Smoke shrimps for 8 minutes, 4 minutes per side. Serve and enjoy.
Nutrition Info: Calories: 267 Cal Fat: 11.6 g Carbohydrates: 4.9 g   Protein: 34.9 g Fiber:0.4 g

132. Wood-fired Halibut

Servings: 4   Cooking Time: 20 Minutes
Ingredients:
- 1 pound halibut fillet
- 1 batch Dill Seafood Rub

Directions:
Supply your smoker with wood pellets and follow the manufacturer's specific start-up procedure. Preheat the grill, with the lid closed, to 325°F.   Sprinkle the halibut fillet on all sides with the rub. Using your hands, work the rub into the meat.   Place the halibut directly on the grill grate and grill until its internal temperature reaches 145°F. Remove the halibut from the grill and serve immediately.

133. Lobster Tail

Servings: 2   Cooking Time: 15 Minutes
Ingredients:
- 10 oz lobster tail
- 1/4 tbsp old bay seasoning
- 1/4 tbsp Himalayan salt
- 2 tbsp butter, melted
- 1 tbsp fresh parsley, chopped

Directions:
Preheat your   to 450F.   Slice the tail down the middle then season it with bay seasoning and salt.   Place the tails directly on the grill with the meat side down. Grill for 15 minutes or until the internal temperature reaches 140F.   Remove from the   and drizzle with butter. Serve when hot garnished with parsley.
Nutrition Info: Calories 305, Total fat 14g, Saturated fat 8g, Total carbs 5g, Net carbs 5g Protein 38g, Sugars 0g, Fiber 0g, Sodium 684mg

134. Bbq Oysters

Servings: 4-6   Cooking Time: 16 Minutes
Ingredients:
- Shucked oysters - 12
- Unsalted butter - 1 lb.
- Chopped green onions - 1 bunch
- Honey Hog BBQ Rub or Meat Church "The Gospel" - 1 tbsp
- Minced green onions - ½ bunch
- Seasoned breadcrumbs - ½ cup
- Cloves of minced garlic - 2
- Shredded pepper jack cheese - 8 oz
- Heat and Sweet BBQ sauce

Directions:
Preheat the pellet grill for about 10-15 minutes with the lid closed.   To make the compound butter, wait for the butter to soften. Then combine the butter, onions, BBQ rub, and garlic thoroughly.   Lay the butter evenly on plastic wrap or parchment paper. Roll it up in a log shape and tie the ends with butcher's twine. Place these in the freezer to solidify for an hour. This butter can be used on any kind of grilled meat to enhance its flavor. Any other high-quality butter can also replace this compound butter.   Shuck the oysters, keeping the juice in the shell. Sprinkle all the oysters with breadcrumbs and place them directly on the grill. Allow them to cook for 5 minutes. You will know they are cooked when the oysters begin to curl slightly at the edges.   Once they are cooked, put a spoonful of the compound butter on the oysters. Once the butter melts, you can add a little bit of pepper jack cheese to add more flavor to them.   The oysters must not be on the grill for longer than 6 minutes, or you risk overcooking them. Put a generous squirt of the BBQ sauce on all the oysters. Also, add a few chopped onions.   Allow them to cool for a few minutes and enjoy the taste of the sea!
Nutrition Info: Carbohydrates: 2.5 g Protein: 4.7 g Fat: 1.1 g Sodium: 53 mg   Cholesterol: 25 mg

135. Grilled Rainbow Trout

Servings: 6   Cooking Time: 2 Hours
Ingredients:
- 6 rainbow trout, cleaned, butterfly
- For the Brine:
- 1/4 cup salt
- 1 tablespoon ground black pepper
- 1/2 cup brown sugar
- 2 tablespoons soy sauce
- 16 cups water

Directions:
Prepare the brine and for this, take a large container, add all of its ingredients in it, stir until sugar has dissolved, then add trout and let soak for 1 hour in the refrigerator. When ready to cook, switch on the   grill, fill the grill hopper with oak flavored wood pellets, power the grill on by using the   control panel, select 'smoke' on the temperature dial, or set the temperature to 225 degrees F and let it preheat for a minimum of 15 minutes. Meanwhile, remove trout from the brine and pat dry with paper towels.   When the grill has preheated, open the lid, place trout on the grill grate, shut the grill and smoke for 2 hours until thoroughly cooked and tender. When done, transfer trout to a dish and then serve.

Nutrition Info: Calories: 250 Cal ;Fat: 12 g ;Carbs: 1.4 g ;Protein: 33 g ;Fiber: 0.3 g

136. Halibut

Servings: 4   Cooking Time: 30 Minutes
Ingredients:
- 1-pound fresh halibut filet (cut into 4 equal sizes)
- 1 tbsp fresh lemon juice
- 2 garlic cloves (minced)
- 2 tsp soy sauce
- ½ tsp ground black pepper
- ½ tsp onion powder
- 2 tbsp honey
- ½ tsp oregano
- 1 tsp dried basil
- 2 tbsp butter (melted)
- Maple syrup for serving

Directions:
Combine the lemon juice, honey, soy sauce, onion powder, oregano, dried basil, pepper and garlic. Brush the halibut filets generously with the filet the mixture. Wrap the filets with aluminum foil and refrigerate for 4 hours.   Remove the filets from the refrigerator and let them sit for about 2 hours, or until they are at room temperature.   Activate your wood pellet grill on smoke, leaving the lid opened for 5 minutes or until fire starts.   The lid must not be opened for it to be preheated and reach 275°F 15 minutes, using fruit wood pellets.   Place the halibut filets directly on the grill grate and smoke for 30 minutes   Remove the filets from the grill and let them rest for 10 minutes.   Serve and top with maple syrup to taste

Nutrition Info: Calories: 180 Cal Fat: 6.3 g
Carbohydrates: 10 g   Protein: 20.6 g Fiber: 0.3 g

137. Lobster Tails

Servings: 4   Cooking Time: 35 Minutes
Ingredients:
- 2 lobster tails, each about 10 ounces
- For the Sauce:
- 2 tablespoons chopped parsley
- 1/4 teaspoon garlic salt
- 1 teaspoon paprika
- 1/4 teaspoon ground black pepper
- 1/4 teaspoon old bay seasoning
- 8 tablespoons butter, unsalted
- 2 tablespoons lemon juice

Directions:
Switch on the   grill, fill the grill hopper with flavored wood pellets, power the grill on by using the control panel, select 'smoke' on the temperature dial, or set the temperature to 450 degrees F and let it preheat for a minimum of 15 minutes.   Meanwhile, prepare the sauce and for this, take a small saucepan, place it over medium-low heat, add butter in it and when it melts, add remaining ingredients for the sauce and stir until combined, set aside until required.   Prepare the lobster and for this, cut the shell from the middle to the tail by using kitchen shears and then take the meat from the shell, keeping it attached at the base of the crab tail. Then butterfly the crab meat by making a slit down the middle, then place lobster tails on a baking sheet and pour 1 tablespoon of sauce over each lobster tail, reserve the remaining sauce.   When the grill has preheated, open the lid, place crab tails on the grill grate, shut the grill and smoke for 30 minutes until opaque.   When done, transfer lobster tails to a dish and then serve with the remaining sauce.

Nutrition Info: Calories: 290 Cal ;Fat: 22 g ;Carbs: 1 g ;Protein: 20 g ;Fiber: 0.3 g

138. Grilled Lobster Tail

Servings: 4   Cooking Time: 15 Minutes
Ingredients:
- 2 (8 ounces each) lobster tails
- 1/4 tsp old bay seasoning
- ½ tsp oregano
- 1 tsp paprika
- Juice from one lemon
- 1/4 tsp Himalayan salt
- 1/4 tsp freshly ground black pepper
- 1/4 tsp onion powder
- 2 tbsp freshly chopped parsley
- 1/4 cup melted butter

Directions:
Slice the tail in the middle with a kitchen shear. Pull the shell apart slightly and run your hand through the meat to separate the meat partially   Combine the seasonings   Drizzle lobster tail with lemon juice and season generously with the seasoning mixture. Preheat your wood pellet smoker to 450°F, using apple wood pellets.   Place the lobster tail directly on the grill grate, meat side down. Cook for about 15 minutes.

The tails must be pulled off and it must cool down for a few minutes   Drizzle melted butter over the tails. Serve and garnish with fresh chopped parsley.
Nutrition Info: Calories: 146 Cal Fat: 11.7 g Carbohydrates: 2.1 g   Protein: 9.3 g Fiber: 0.8 g

139. Oysters In The Shell

Servings: 4   Cooking Time: 20 Minutes
Ingredients:
- 8 medium oysters, unopened, in the shell, rinsed and scrubbed
- 1 batch Lemon Butter Mop for Seafood

Directions:
Supply your smoker with wood pellets and follow the manufacturer's specific start-up procedure. Preheat the grill, with the lid closed, to 375°F.   Place the unopened oysters directly on the grill grate and grill for about 20 minutes, or until the oysters are done and their shells open.   Discard any oysters that do not open. Shuck the remaining oysters, transfer them to a bowl, and add the mop. Serve immediately.

140. Wood Pellet Rockfish

Servings: 6   Cooking Time: 20 Minutes
Ingredients:
- 6 rockfish fillets
- 1 lemon, sliced
- 3/4 tbsp Himalayan salt
- 2 tbsp fresh dill, chopped
- 1/2 tbsp garlic powder
- 1/2 tbsp onion powder
- 6 tbsp butter

Directions:
Preheat your wood pellet grill to 375°F.   Place the rockfish in a baking dish and season with salt, dill, garlic, and onion.   Place butter on top of the fish then close the lid. Cook for 20 minutes or until the fish is no longer translucent.   Remove from grill and let sit for 5 minutes before serving. enjoy.
Nutrition Info: Calories 270, Total fat 17g, Saturated fat 9g, Total Carbs 2g, Net Carbs 0g, Protein 28g, Sugar 0g, Fiber 0g, Sodium: 381mg

141. Stuffed Shrimp Tilapia

Servings: 5   Cooking Time: 45 Minutes
Ingredients:
- 5 ounces fresh, farmed tilapia fillets
- 2 tablespoons extra virgin olive oil
- 1and ½ teaspoons smoked paprika
- 1and ½ teaspoons Old Bay seasoning
- Shrimp stuffing
- 1pound shrimp, cooked and deveined
- 1tablespoon salted butter
- 1cup red onion, diced
- 1cup Italian bread crumbs
- ½ cup mayonnaise

- 1large egg, beaten
- 2teaspoons fresh parsley, chopped
- 1and ½ teaspoons salt and pepper

Directions:
Take a food processor and add shrimp, chop them up   Take a skillet and place it over medium-high heat, add butter and allow it to melt   Sauté the onions for 3 minutes   Add chopped shrimp with cooled Sautéed onion alongside remaining ingredients listed under stuffing ingredients and transfer to a bowl   Cover the mixture and allow it to refrigerate for 60 minutes   Rub both sides of the fillet with olive oil   Spoon 1/3 cup of the stuffing to the fillet   Flatten out the stuffing onto the bottom half of the fillet and fold the Tilapia in half   Secure with 2 toothpicks   Dust each fillet with smoked paprika and Old Bay seasoning   Preheat your smoker to 400 degrees Fahrenheit   Add your preferred wood Pellets and transfer the fillets to a non-stick grill tray   Transfer to your smoker and smoker for 30-45 minutes until the internal temperature reaches 145 degrees Fahrenheit   Allow the fish to rest for 5 minutes and enjoy!
Nutrition Info: Calories: 620 Fats: 50g Carbs: 6g Fiber: 1g

142. Wine Infused Salmon

Servings: 4   Cooking Time: 5 Hours
Ingredients:
- 2 C. low-sodium soy sauce
- 1 C. dry white wine
- 1 C. water
- ½ tsp. Tabasco sauce
- 1/3 C. sugar
- ¼ C. salt
- ½ tsp. garlic powder
- ½ tsp. onion powder
- Freshly ground black pepper, to taste
- 4 (6-oz.) salmon fillets

Directions:
In a large bowl, add all ingredients except salmon and stir until sugar is dissolved.   Add salmon fillets and coat with brine well.   Refrigerate, covered overnight. Remove salmon from bowl and rinse under cold running water.   With paper towels, pat dry the salmon fillets. Arrange a wire rack in a sheet pan.   Place the salmon fillets onto wire rack, skin side down and set aside to cool for about 1 hour.   Set the temperature of Grill to 165 degrees F and preheat with closed lid for 15 minutes, using charcoal.   Place the salmon fillets onto the grill, skin side down and cook for about 3-5 hours or until desired doneness.   Remove the salmon fillets from grill and serve hot.
Nutrition Info: Calories per serving: 377; Carbohydrates: 26.3g; Protein: 41.1g; Fat: 10.5g; Sugar: 25.1g; Sodium: 14000mg; Fiber: 0g

143. Pacific Northwest Salmon

Servings: 4   Cooking Time: 1 Hour, 15 Minutes

Ingredients:
- 1 (2-pound) half salmon fillet
- 1 batch Dill Seafood Rub
- 2 tablespoons butter, cut into 3 or 4 slices

Directions:
Supply your smoker with wood pellets and follow the manufacturer's specific start-up procedure. Preheat the grill, with the lid closed, to 180°F.   Season the salmon all over with the rub. Using your hands, work the rub into the flesh.   Place the salmon directly on the grill grate, skin-side down, and smoke for 1 hour.   Place the butter slices on the salmon, equally spaced. Increase the grill's temperature to 300°F and continue to cook until the salmon's internal temperature reaches 145°F. Remove the salmon from the grill and serve immediately.

144. Grilled Tuna

Servings: 4   Cooking Time: 4 Minutes

Ingredients:
- 4 (6 ounce each) tuna steaks (1 inch thick)
- 1 lemon (juiced)
- 1 clove garlic (minced)
- 1 tsp chili
- 2 tbsp extra virgin olive oil
- 1 cup white wine
- 3 tbsp brown sugar
- 1 tsp rosemary

Directions:
Combine lemon, chili, white wine, sugar, rosemary, olive oil and garlic. Add the tuna steaks and toss to combine. Transfer the tuna and marinade to a zip-lock bag. Refrigerate for 3 hours.   Remove the tuna steaks from the marinade and let them rest for about 1 hour   Start your grill on smoke, leaving the lid opened for 5 minutes, or until fire starts.   Do not open lid to preheat until 15 minutes to the setting "HIGH"   Grease the grill grate with oil and place the tuna on the grill grate. Grill tuna steaks for 4 minutes, 2 minutes per side.   Remove the tuna from the grill and let them rest for a few minutes.

Nutrition Info: Calories: 137 Cal Fat: 17.8 g Carbohydrates: 10.2 g   Protein: 51.2 g Fiber: 0.6 g

145. Summer Paella

Servings: 6   Cooking Time: 45 Minutes

Ingredients:
- 6 tablespoons extra-virgin olive oil, divided, plus more for drizzling
- 2 green or red bell peppers, cored, seeded, and diced
- 2 medium onions, diced
- 2 garlic cloves, slivered
- 1 (29-ounce) can tomato purée
- 1½ pounds chicken thighs
- Kosher salt
- 1½ pounds tail-on shrimp, peeled and deveined
- 1 cup dried thinly sliced chorizo sausage
- 1 tablespoon smoked paprika
- 1½ teaspoons saffron threads

- 2 quarts chicken broth
- 3½ cups white rice
- 2 (7½-ounce) cans chipotle chiles in adobo sauce
- 1½ pounds fresh clams, soaked in cold water for 15 to 20 minutes2 tablespoons chopped fresh parsley
- 2 lemons, cut into wedges, for serving

Directions:
Make the sofrito: On the stove top, in a saucepan over medium-low heat, combine ¼ cup of olive oil, the bell peppers, onions, and garlic, and cook for 5 minutes, or until the onions are translucent.   Stir in the tomato purée, reduce the heat to low, and simmer, stirring frequently, until most of the liquid has evaporated, about 30 minutes. Set aside. (Note: The sofrito can be made in advance and refrigerated.)   Supply your smoker with wood pellets and follow the manufacturer's specific start-up procedure. Preheat, with the lid closed, to 450°F. Heat a large paella pan on the smoker and add the remaining 2 tablespoons of olive oil.   Add the chicken thighs, season lightly with salt, and brown for 6 to 10 minutes, then push to the outer edge of the pan.   Add the shrimp, season with salt, close the lid, and smoke for 3 minutes.   Add the sofrito, chorizo, paprika, and saffron, and stir together.   In a separate bowl, combine the chicken broth, uncooked rice, and 1 tablespoon of salt, stirring until well combined.   Add the broth-rice mixture to the paella pan, spreading it evenly over the other ingredients.   Close the lid and smoke for 5 minutes, then add the chipotle chiles and clams on top of the rice.   Close the lid and continue to smoke the paella for about 30 minutes, or until all of the liquid is absorbed. Remove the pan from the grill, cover tightly with aluminum foil, and let rest off the heat for 5 minutes. Drizzle with olive oil, sprinkle with the fresh parsley, and serve with the lemon wedges.

146. Blackened Salmon

Servings: 4   Cooking Time: 30 Minutes

Ingredients:
- 2 lb. salmon, fillet, scaled and deboned
- 2 tablespoons olive oil
- 4 tablespoons sweet dry rub
- 1 tablespoon cayenne pepper
- 2 cloves garlic, minced

Directions:
Turn on your wood pellet grill.   Set it to 350 degrees F. Brush the salmon with the olive oil.   Sprinkle it with the dry rub, cayenne pepper, and garlic.   Grill for 5 minutes per side.

Nutrition Info: Calories: 460Fat: 23 gCholesterol: 140 mgCarbohydrates: 7 g Fiber: 5 g Sugars: 2 g Protein: 50 g

147. Wood Pellet Grilled Lobster Tail

Servings: 2   Cooking Time: 15 Minutes

Ingredients:
- 10 oz lobster tail

- 1/4 tbsp old bay seasoning
- 1/4 tbsp Himalayan sea salt
- 2 tbsp butter, melted
- 1 tbsp fresh parsley, chopped

Directions:
Preheat the wood pellet to 450°F.   Slice the tails down the middle using a knife.   Season with seasoning and salt then place the tails on the grill grate.   Grill for 15 minutes or until the internal temperature reaches 140°F.. Remove the tails and drizzle with butter and garnish with parsley.   Serve and enjoy.

Nutrition Info: Calories 305, Total fat 14g, Saturated fat 8g, Total Carbs 5g, Net Carbs 5g, Protein 18g, Sugar 0g, Fiber 0g, Sodium: 685mg, Potassium 159mg

148. Spicy Shrimp

Servings: 4   Cooking Time: 10 Minutes
Ingredients:
- 3 tablespoons olive oil
- 6 cloves garlic
- 2 tablespoons chicken dry rub
- 6 oz. chili
- 1 1/2 tablespoons white vinegar
- 1 1/2 teaspoons sugar
- 2 lb. shrimp, peeled and deveined

Directions:
Add olive oil, garlic, dry rub, chili, vinegar and sugar in a food processor.   Blend until smooth.   Transfer mixture to a bowl.   Stir in shrimp.   Cover and refrigerate for 30 minutes.   Preheat the wood pellet grill to hit for 15 minutes while the lid is closed. Thread shrimp onto skewers.   Grill for 3 minute per side.   Tips: You can also add vegetables to the skewers.

149. No-fuss Tuna Burgers

Servings: 6   Cooking Time: 15 Minutes
Ingredients:
- 2 lb. tuna steak
- 1 green bell pepper, seeded and chopped
- 1 white onion, chopped
- 2 eggs
- 1 tsp. soy sauce
- 1 tbsp. blackened Saskatchewan rub
- Salt and freshly ground black pepper, to taste

Directions:
Set the temperature of Grill to 500 degrees F and preheat with closed lid for 15 minutes.   In a bowl, add all the ingredients and mix until well combined.   With greased hands, make patties from mixture.   Place the patties onto the grill close to the edges and cook for about 10-15 minutes, flipping once halfway through.   Serve hot.

Nutrition Info: Calories per serving: 313; Carbohydrates: 3.4g; Protein: 47.5g; Fat: 11g; Sugar: 1.9g; Sodium: 174mg; Fiber: 0.7g

150. Blackened Catfish

Servings: 4   Cooking Time: 40 Minutes
Ingredients:
- Spice blend
- 1teaspoon granulated garlic
- 1/4 teaspoon cayenne pepper
- 1/2 cup Cajun seasoning
- 1teaspoon ground thyme
- 1teaspoon ground oregano
- 1teaspoon onion powder
- 1tablespoon smoked paprika
- 1teaspoon pepper
- Fish
- 4 catfish fillets
- Salt to taste
- 1/2 cup butter

Directions:
In a bowl, combine all the ingredients for the spice blend. Sprinkle both sides of the fish with the salt and spice blend.   Set your wood pellet grill to 450 degrees F. Heat your cast iron pan and add the butter. Add the fillets to the pan.   Cook for 5 minutes per side.   Serving Suggestion: Garnish with lemon wedges.   Tip: Smoke the catfish for 20 minutes before seasoning.

Nutrition Info: Calories: 181.5 Fat: 10.5 g Cholesterol: 65.8 mg Carbohydrates: 2.9 g Fiber: 1.8 g Sugars: 0.4 g Protein: 19.2 g

151. Sriracha Salmon

Servings: 4   Cooking Time: 25 Minutes
Ingredients:
- 3-pound salmon, skin on
- For the Marinade:
- 1 teaspoon lime zest
- 1 tablespoon minced garlic
- 1 tablespoon grated ginger
- Sea salt as needed
- Ground black pepper as needed
- 1/4 cup maple syrup
- 2 tablespoons soy sauce
- 2 tablespoons Sriracha sauce
- 1 tablespoon toasted sesame oil
- 1 tablespoon rice vinegar
- 1 teaspoon toasted sesame seeds

Directions:
Prepare the marinade and for this, take a small bowl, place all of its ingredients in it, stir until well combined, and then pour the mixture into a large plastic bag. Add salmon in the bag, seal it, turn it upside down to coat salmon with the marinade and let it marinate for a minimum of 2 hours in the refrigerator.   When ready to cook, switch on the grill, fill the grill hopper with flavored wood pellets, power the grill on by using the control panel, select 'smoke' on the temperature dial, or set the temperature to 450 degrees F and let it preheat for a minimum of 5 minutes.   Meanwhile, take a large baking sheet, line it with parchment paper, place salmon on it skin-side down and then brush with the marinade.

When the grill has preheated, open the lid, place baking sheet containing salmon on the grill grate, shut the grill and smoke for 25 minutes until thoroughly cooked. When done, transfer salmon to a dish and then serve.
Nutrition Info: Calories: 360 Cal ;Fat: 21 g ;Carbs: 28 g ;Protein: 16 g ;Fiber: 1.5 g

152. Wood Pellet Garlic Dill Smoked Salmon

Servings: 12   Cooking Time: 4 Hours
Ingredients:
- 2 salmon fillets
- Brine
- 4 cups water
- 1 cup brown sugar
- 1/3 cup kosher salt
- Seasoning
- 3 tbsp minced garlic
- 1 tbsp fresh dill, chopped

Directions:
In a zip lock bag, combine the brine ingredients until all sugar has dissolved. Place the salmon in the bag and refrigerate overnight.   Remove the salmon from the brine, rinse with water and pat dry with a paper towel. Let it rest for 2-4 hours at room temperature.   Season the salmon with garlic and dill generously.   Fire up the wood pellet grill to smoke and place the salmon on a cooling rack that is coated with cooking spray.   Place the rack in the smoker and close the lid.   Smoke the salmon for 4 hours until the smoke is between 130-180°F. Remove the salmon from the grill and serve with crackers. Enjoy
Nutrition Info: Calories 139, Total fat 5g, Saturated fat 1g, Total Carbs 16g, Net Carbs 16g, Protein 9g, Sugar 0g, Fiber 0g, Sodium: 3143mg

153. Grilled Teriyaki Salmon

Servings: 4   Cooking Time: 30 Minutes
Ingredients:
- 1 salmon fillet
- 1/8 cup olive oil
- 1/2 tbsp salt
- 1/4 tbsp pepper
- 1/4 tbsp garlic salt
- 1/4 cup butter, sliced
- 1/4 teriyaki sauce
- 1 tbsp sesame seeds

Directions:
Preheat the grill to 400°F.   Place the salmon fillet on a non-stick foil sheet. Drizzle the salmon with oil, seasonings, and butter on top.   Pace the foil tray on the grill and close the lid. Cook for 8 minutes then open the lid.   Brush the salmon with teriyaki sauce and repeat after every 5 minutes until all sauce is finished. The internal temperature should be 145°F.   Remove the salmon from the grill and sprinkle with sesame seeds. Serve and enjoy with your favorite side dish.

Nutrition Info: Calories 296, Total fat 25g, Saturated fat 10g, Total Carbs 3g, Net Carbs 3g, Protein 14g, Sugar 3g, Fiber 0g, Sodium: 1179mg, Potassium 459mg

154. Crab Stuffed Lingcod

Servings: 6   Cooking Time: 30 Minutes
Ingredients:
- Lemon cream sauce
- 4 garlic cloves
- 1 shallot
- 1 leek
- 2 tbsp olive oil
- 1 tbsp salt
- 1/4 tbsp black pepper
- 3 tbsp butter
- 1/4 cup white wine
- 1 cup whipping cream
- 2 tbsp lemon juice
- 1 tbsp lemon zest
- Crab mix
- 1 lb crab meat
- 1/3 cup mayo
- 1/3 cup sour cream
- 1/3 cup lemon cream sauce
- 1/4 green onion, chopped
- 1/4 tbsp black pepper
- 1/2 tbsp old bay seasoning
- Fish
- 2 lb lingcod
- 1 tbsp olive oil
- 1 tbsp salt
- 1 tbsp paprika
- 1 tbsp green onion, chopped
- 1 tbsp Italian parsley

Directions:
Lemon cream sauce   Chop garlic, shallot, and leeks then add to a saucepan with oil, salt, pepper, and butter. Saute over medium heat until the shallot is translucent. Deglaze with white wine then add whipping cream. Bring the sauce to boil, reduce heat and simmer for 3 minutes.   Remove from heat and add lemon juice and lemon zest. Transfer the sauce to a blender and blend until smooth.   Set aside 1/3 cup for the crab mix Crab mix   Add all the ingredients in a mixing bowl and mix thoroughly until well combined.   Set aside   Fish Fire up your   to high heat then slice the fish into 6-ounce portions.   Lay the fish on its side on a cutting board and slice it 3/4 way through the middle leaving a 1/2 inch on each end so as to have a nice pouch.   Rub the oil into the fish then place them on a baking sheet. Sprinkle with salt.   Stuff crab mix into each fish then sprinkle paprika and place it on the grill.   Cook for 15 minutes or more if the fillets are more than 2 inches thick. Remove the fish and transfer to serving platters. Pour the remaining lemon cream sauce on each fish and garnish with onions and parsley.
Nutrition Info: Calories 476, Total fat 33g, Saturated fat 14g, Total carbs 6g, Net carbs 5g Protein 38g, Sugars 3g, Fiber 1g, Sodium 1032mg

155. Cider Salmon

Servings: 4   Cooking Time: 1 Hour

Ingredients:
- 1 ½ pound salmon fillet, skin-on, center-cut, pin bone removed
- For the Brine:
- 4 juniper berries, crushed
- 1 bay leaf, crumbled
- 1 piece star anise, broken
- 1 1/2 cups apple cider
- For the Cure:
- 1/2 cup salt
- 1 teaspoon ground black pepper
- 1/4 cup brown sugar
- 2 teaspoons barbecue rub

Directions:
Prepare the brine and for this, take a large container, add all of its ingredients in it, stir until mixed, then add salmon and let soak for a minimum of 8 hours in the refrigerator.   Meanwhile, prepare the cure and for this, take a small bowl, place all of its ingredients in it and stir until combined.   After 8 hours, remove salmon from the brine, then take a baking dish, place half of the cure in it, top with salmon skin-side down, sprinkle remaining cure on top, cover with plastic wrap and let it rest for 1 hour in the refrigerator.   When ready to cook, switch on the   grill, fill the grill hopper with oak flavored wood pellets, power the grill on by using the control panel, select 'smoke' on the temperature dial, or set the temperature to 200 degrees F and let it preheat for a minimum of 5 minutes.   Meanwhile, remove salmon from the cure, pat dry with paper towels, and then sprinkle with black pepper.   When the grill has preheated, open the lid, place salmon on the grill grate, shut the grill, and smoke for 1 hour until the internal temperature reaches 150 degrees F.   When done, transfer salmon to a cutting board, let it rest for 5 minutes, then remove the skin and serve.

Nutrition Info: Calories: 233 Cal ;Fat: 14 g ;Carbs: 0 g ;Protein: 25 g ;Fiber: 0 g

156. Wood Pellet Smoked Buffalo Shrimp

Servings: 6   Cooking Time: 5 Minutes

Ingredients:
- 1 lb raw shrimps peeled and deveined
- 1/2 tbsp salt
- 1/4 tbsp garlic salt
- 1/4 tbsp garlic powder
- 1/4 tbsp onion powder
- 1/2 cup buffalo sauce

Directions:
Preheat the wood pellet grill to 450°F.   Coat the shrimp with both salts, garlic and onion powders. Place the shrimp in a grill and cook for 3 minutes on each side.   Remove from the grill and toss in buffalo sauce. Serve with cheese, celery and napkins. Enjoy.

Nutrition Info: Calories 57, Total fat 1g, Saturated fat 0g, Total Carbs 1g, Net Carbs 1g, Protein 10g, Sugar 0g, Fiber 0g, Sodium: 1106mg, Potassium 469mg.

157. Salmon With Avocado Salsa

Servings: 6   Cooking Time: 20 Minutes

Ingredients:
- 3 lb. salmon fillet
- Garlic salt and pepper to taste
- 4 cups avocado, sliced into cubes
- 1 onion, chopped
- 1 jalapeño pepper, minced
- 1 tablespoon lime juice
- 1 tablespoon olive oil
- ¼ cup cilantro, chopped
- Salt to taste

Directions:
Sprinkle both sides of salmon with garlic salt and pepper. Set the   wood pellet grill to smoke.   Grill the salmon for 7 to 8 minutes per side.   While waiting, prepare the salsa by combining the remaining ingredients in a bowl. Serve salmon with the avocado salsa.   Tips: You can also use tomato salsa for this recipe if you don't have avocados.

158. Grilled Shrimp Kabobs

Servings: 4   Cooking Time: 10 Minutes

Ingredients:
- 1 lb. colossal shrimp, peeled and deveined
- 2 tbsp. oil
- 1/2 tbsp. garlic salt
- 1/2 tbsp. salt
- 1/8 tbsp. pepper
- 6 skewers

Directions:
Preheat your   to 375F.   Pat the shrimp dry with a paper towel.   In a mixing bowl, mix oil, garlic salt, salt, and pepper   Toss the shrimp in the mixture until well coated.   Skewer the shrimps and cook in the   with the lid closed for 4 minutes.   Open the lid, flip the skewers and cook for another 4 minutes or until the shrimp is pink and the flesh is opaque.   Serve.

Nutrition Info: Calories 325, Total fat 0g, Saturated fat 0g, Total carbs 0g, Net carbs 0g Protein 20g, Sugars 0g, Fiber 0g, Sodium 120mg

159. Octopus With Lemon And Oregano

Servings: 4   Cooking Time: 1 Hour And 30 Minutes

Ingredients:
- 3 lemons
- 3 pounds cleaned octopus, thawed if frozen
- 6 cloves garlic, peeled
- 4 sprigs fresh oregano
- 2 bay leaves
- Salt and pepper
- 3 tablespoons good-quality olive oil

- Minced fresh oregano for garnish

Directions:
Halve one of the lemons. Put the octopus, garlic, oregano sprigs, bay leaves, a large pinch of salt, and lemon halves in a large pot with enough water to cover by a couple of inches. Bring to a boil, adjust the heat so the liquid bubbles gently but steadily, and cook, occasionally turning with tongs, until the octopus is tender 30 to 90 minutes. (Check with the tip of a sharp knife; it should go in smoothly.) Drain; discard the seasonings. (You can cover and refrigerate the octopus for up to 24 hours.) Start the coals or heat a gas grill for direct hot cooking. Make sure the grates are clean.   Squeeze the juice 1 of the remaining lemons and whisk it with the oil and salt and pepper to taste. Cut the octopus into large serving pieces and toss with the oil mixture.   Put the octopus on the grill directly over the fire. Cover the grill and cook until heated through and charred, 4 to 5 minutes per side. Cut the remaining lemon in wedges. Transfer the octopus to a platter, sprinkle with minced oregano, and serve with the lemon wedges.

Nutrition Info: Calories: 139 Fats: 1.8 g Cholesterol: 0 mg Carbohydrates: 3.7 g Fiber: 0 g Sugars: 0 g Proteins: 25.4 g

160. Grilled Lingcod

Servings: 6   Cooking Time: 15 Minutes
Ingredients:
- 2 lb lingcod fillets
- 1/2 tbsp salt
- 1/2 tbsp white pepper
- 1/4 tbsp cayenne
- Lemon wedges

Directions:
Preheat the wood pellet grill to 375°F.   Place the lingcod on a parchment paper and season it with salt, white pepper, cayenne pepper then top with the lemon. Place the fish on the grill and cook for 15 minutes or until the internal temperature reaches 145°F.   Serve and enjoy.

Nutrition Info: Calories 245, Total fat 2g, Saturated fat 0g, Total Carbs 2g, Net Carbs 1g, Protein 52g, Sugar 1g, Fiber 1g, Sodium: 442mg, Potassium 649mg

161. Mango Shrimp

Servings: 4   Cooking Time: 15 Minutes
Ingredients:
- 1lb. shrimp, peeled and deveined but tail intact
- 2tablespoons olive oil
- Mango seasoning

Directions:
Turn on your wood pellet grill.   Preheat it to 425 degrees F.   Coat the shrimp with the oil and season with the mango seasoning.   Thread the shrimp into skewers.   Grill for 3 minutes per side.   Serving Suggestion: Garnish with chopped parsley.

Nutrition Info: Calories: 223.1 Fat: 4.3 g Cholesterol: 129.2 mg Carbohydrates: 29.2 g Fiber: 4.4 g Sugars: 15.6g Protein: 19.5 g

162. Grilled Blackened Salmon

Servings: 4   Cooking Time: 30 Minutes
Ingredients:
- 4 salmon fillet
- Blackened dry rub
- Italian seasoning powder

Directions:
Season salmon fillets with dry rub and seasoning powder. Grill in the   wood pellet grill at 325 degrees F for 10 to 15 minutes per side.   Tips: You can also drizzle salmon with lemon juice

163. Flavor-bursting Prawn Skewers

Servings: 5   Cooking Time: 8 Minutes
Ingredients:
- ¼ C. fresh parsley leaves, minced
- 1 tbsp. garlic, crushed
- 2½ tbsp. olive oil
- 2 tbsp. Thai chili sauce
- 1 tbsp. fresh lime juice
- 1½ pounds prawns, peeled and deveined

Directions:
In a large bowl, add all ingredients except for prawns and mix well.   In a resealable plastic bag, add marinade and prawns.   Seal the bag and shake to coat well Refrigerate for   about 20-30 minutes.   Set the temperature of   Grill to 450 degrees F and preheat with closed lid for 15 minutes.   Remove the prawns from marinade and thread onto metal skewers.   Arrange the skewers onto the grill and cook for about 4 minutes per side.   Remove the skewers from grill and serve hot.

Nutrition Info: Calories per serving: 234; Carbohydrates: 4.9g; Protein: 31.2g; Fat: 9.3g; Sugar: 1.7g; Sodium: 562mg; Fiber: 0.1g

164. Halibut In Parchment

Servings: 4   Cooking Time: 15 Minutes
Ingredients:
- 16 asparagus spears, trimmed, sliced into 1/2-inch pieces
- 2 ears of corn kernels
- 4 ounces halibut fillets, pin bones removed
- 2 lemons, cut into 12 slices
- Salt as needed
- Ground black pepper as needed
- 2 tablespoons olive oil
- 2 tablespoons chopped parsley

Directions:
Switch on the   grill, fill the grill hopper with flavored wood pellets, power the grill on by using the control panel, select 'smoke' on the temperature dial, or set the temperature to 450 degrees F and let it preheat for a

minimum of 5 minutes. Meanwhile, cut out 18-inch long parchment paper, place a fillet in the center of each parchment, season with salt and black pepper, and then drizzle with oil. Cover each fillet with three lemon slices, overlapping slightly, sprinkle one-fourth of asparagus and corn on each fillet, season with some salt and black pepper, and seal the fillets and vegetables tightly to prevent steam from escaping the packet. When the grill has preheated, open the lid, place fillet packets on the grill grate, shut the grill and smoke for 15 minutes until packets have turned slightly brown and puffed up. When done, transfer packets to a dish, let them stand for 5 minutes, then cut 'X' in the center of each packet, carefully uncover the fillets an vegetables, sprinkle with parsley, and then serve.

Nutrition Info: Calories: 186.6 Cal ;Fat: 2.8 g ;Carbs: 14.2 g ;Protein: 25.7 g ;Fiber: 4.1 g

165. Enticing Mahi-mahi

Servings: 4   Cooking Time: 10 Minutes
Ingredients:
- 4 (6-oz.) mahi-mahi fillets
- 2 tbsp. olive oil
- Salt and freshly ground black pepper, to taste

Directions:
Set the temperature of Grill to 350 degrees F and preheat with closed lid for 15 minutes. Coat fish fillets with olive oil and season with salt and black pepper evenly. Place the fish fillets onto the grill and cook for about 5 minutes per side. Remove the fish fillets from grill and serve hot.

Nutrition Info: Calories per serving: 195; Carbohydrates: 0g; Protein: 31.6g; Fat: 7g; Sugar: 0g; Sodium: 182mg; Fiber: 0g

166. Cajun-blackened Shrimp

Servings: 4   Cooking Time: 20 Minutes
Ingredients:
- 1 pound peeled and deveined shrimp, with tails on
- 1 batch Cajun Rub
- 8 tablespoons (1 stick) butter
- ¼ cup Worcestershire sauce

Directions:
Supply your smoker with wood pellets and follow the manufacturer's specific start-up procedure. Preheat the grill, with the lid closed, to 450°F and place a cast-iron skillet on the grill grate. Wait about 10 minutes after your grill has reached temperature, allowing the skillet to get hot. Meanwhile, season the shrimp all over with the rub. When the skillet is hot, place the butter in it to melt. Once the butter melts, stir in the Worcestershire sauce. Add the shrimp and gently stir to coat. Smoke-braise the shrimp for about 10 minutes per side, until opaque and cooked through. Remove the shrimp from the grill and serve immediately.

167. Lively Flavored Shrimp

Servings: 6   Cooking Time: 30 Minutes
Ingredients:
- 8 oz. salted butter, melted
- ¼ C. Worcestershire sauce
- ¼ C. fresh parsley, chopped
- 1 lemon, quartered
- 2 lb. jumbo shrimp, peeled and deveined
- 3 tbsp. BBQ rub

Directions:
In a metal baking pan, add all ingredients except for shrimp and BBQ rub and mix well. Season the shrimp with BBQ rub evenly. Add the shrimp in the pan with butter mixture and coat well. Set aside for about 20-30 minutes. Set the temperature of Grill to 250 degrees F and preheat with closed lid for 15 minutes. Place the pan onto the grill and cook for about 25-30 minutes. Remove the pan from grill and serve hot.

Nutrition Info: Calories per serving: 462; Carbohydrates: 4.7g; Protein: 34.9g; Fat: 33.3g; Sugar: 2.1g; Sodium: 485mg; Fiber: 0.2g

168. Barbecued Scallops

Servings: 4   Cooking Time: 10 Minutes
Ingredients:
- 1 pound large scallops
- 2 tablespoons olive oil
- 1 batch Dill Seafood Rub

Directions:
Supply your smoker with wood pellets and follow the manufacturer's specific start-up procedure. Preheat the grill, with the lid closed, to 375°F. Coat the scallops all over with olive oil and season all sides with the rub. Place the scallops directly on the grill grate and grill for 5 minutes per side. Remove the scallops from the grill and serve immediately.

169. Spicy Shrimps Skewers

Servings: 4   Cooking Time: 6 Minutes
Ingredients:
- 2 pounds shrimp, peeled, and deveined
- For the Marinade:
- 6 ounces Thai chilies
- 6 cloves of garlic, peeled
- 1 ½ teaspoon sugar
- 2 tablespoons Napa Valley rub
- 1 ½ tablespoon white vinegar
- 3 tablespoons olive oil

Directions:
Prepare the marinade and for this, place all of its ingredients in a food processor and then pulse for 1 minute until smooth. Take a large bowl, place shrimps on it, add prepared marinade, toss until well coated, and let marinate for a minimum of 30 minutes in the refrigerator. When ready to cook, switch on the grill, fill the grill hopper with apple-flavored wood pellets, power the grill on by using the control panel, select

'smoke' on the temperature dial, or set the temperature to 450 degrees F and let it preheat for a minimum of 5 minutes. Meanwhile, remove shrimps from the marinade and then thread onto skewers. When the grill has preheated, open the lid, place shrimps' skewers on the grill grate, shut the grill and smoke for 3 minutes per side until firm. When done, transfer shrimps' skewers to a dish and then serve.

Nutrition Info: Calories: 187.2 Cal ;Fat: 2.7 g ;Carbs: 2.7 g ;Protein: 23.2 g ;Fiber: 0.2 g

170. Dijon-smoked Halibut

Servings: 6   Cooking Time: 2 Hours
Ingredients:
- 4 (6-ounce) halibut steaks
- ¼ cup extra-virgin olive oil
- 2 teaspoons kosher salt
- 1 teaspoon freshly ground black pepper
- ½ cup mayonnaise
- ½ cup sweet pickle relish
- ¼ cup finely chopped sweet onion
- ¼ cup chopped roasted red pepper
- ¼ cup finely chopped tomato
- ¼ cup finely chopped cucumber
- 2 tablespoons Dijon mustard
- 1 teaspoon minced garlic

Directions:
Rub the halibut steaks with the olive oil and season on both sides with the salt and pepper. Transfer to a plate, cover with plastic wrap, and refrigerate for 4 hours. Supply your smoker with wood pellets and follow the manufacturer's specific start-up procedure. Preheat, with the lid closed, to 200°F. Remove the halibut from the refrigerator and rub with the mayonnaise. Put the fish directly on the grill grate, close the lid, and smoke for 2 hours, or until opaque and an instant-read thermometer inserted in the fish reads 140°F. While the fish is smoking, combine the pickle relish, onion, roasted red pepper, tomato, cucumber, Dijon mustard, and garlic in a medium bowl. Refrigerate the mustard relish until ready to serve. Serve the halibut steaks hot with the mustard relish.

171. Smoked Shrimp

Servings: 6   Cooking Time: 10 Minutes
Ingredients:
- 1 lb tail-on shrimp, uncooked
- 1/2 tbsp onion powder
- 1/2 tbsp garlic powder
- 1/2 tbsp salt
- 4 tbsp teriyaki sauce
- 2 tbsp green onion, minced
- 4 tbsp sriracha mayo

Directions:
Peel the shrimp shells leaving the tail on then wash well and rise. Drain well and pat dry with a paper towel. Preheat your   to 450F. Season the shrimp with onion powder, garlic powder, and salt. Place the shrimp

in the   and cook for 6 minutes on each side. Remove the shrimp from the   and toss with teriyaki sauce then garnish with onions and mayo.

Nutrition Info: Calories 87, Total fat 0g, Saturated fat 0g, Total carbs 2g, Net carbs 2g Protein 16g, Sugars 0g, Fiber 0g, Sodium 1241mg

172. Grilled Lingcod

Servings: 6   Cooking Time: 15 Minutes
Ingredients:
- 2 lb lingcod fillets
- 1/2 tbsp salt
- 1/2 tbsp white pepper
- 1/4 tbsp cayenne pepper
- Lemon wedges

Directions:
Preheat your   to 375F. Place the lingcod on a parchment paper or on a grill mat   Season the fish with salt, pepper, and top with lemon wedges. Cook the fish for 15 minutes or until the internal temperature reaches 145F.

Nutrition Info: Calories 245, Total fat 2g, Saturated fat 0g, Total carbs 2g, Net carbs 0g Protein 52g, Sugars 1g, Fiber 1g, Sodium 442mg

173. Cajun Catfish

Servings: 6   Cooking Time: 15 Minutes
Ingredients:
- 2½ pounds catfish fillets
- 2 tablespoons olive oil
- 1 batch Cajun Rub

Directions:
Supply your smoker with wood pellets and follow the manufacturer's specific start-up procedure. Preheat the grill, with the lid closed, to 300°F. Coat the catfish fillets all over with olive oil and season with the rub. Using your hands, work the rub into the flesh. Place the fillets directly on the grill grate and smoke until their internal temperature reaches 145°F. Remove the catfish from the grill and serve immediately

174. Wood Pellet Smoked Salmon

Servings: 8   Cooking Time: 4 Hours
Ingredients:
- Brine
- 4 cups water
- 1 cup brown sugar
- 1/3 cup kosher salt
- Salmon
- Salmon fillet, skin in
- Maple syrup

Directions:
Combine all the brine ingredients until the sugar has fully dissolved. Add the brine to a ziplock bag with the salmon and refrigerate for 12 hours. Remove the salmon from the brine, wash it and rinse with water. Pat

dry with paper towel then let sit at room temperature for 2 hours.   Startup your wood pellet to smoke and place the salmon on a baking rack sprayed with cooking spray. After cooking for an hour, baste the salmon with maple syrup. Do not let the smoker get above 180°F for accurate results.   Smoke for 3-4 hours or until the salmon flakes easily.

Nutrition Info: Calories 101, Total fat 2g, Saturated fat 0g, Total carbs 16g, Net carbs 16g, Protein 4g, Sugar 16g, Fiber 0g, Sodium: 3131mg

175. Wood Pellet Salt And Pepper Spot Prawn Skewers

Servings: 6   Cooking Time: 10 Minutes
Ingredients:
- 2 lb spot prawns, clean
- 2 tbsp oil
- Salt and pepper to taste

Directions:
Preheat your grill to 400°F.   Meanwhile, soak the skewers then skewer with the prawns.   Brush with oil then season with salt and pepper to taste.   Place the skewers in the grill, close the lid, and cook for 5 minutes on each side.   Remove from the grill and serve. Enjoy.

Nutrition Info: Calories 221, Total fat 7g, Saturated fat 1g, Total Carbs 2g, Net Carbs 2g, Protein 34g, Sugar 0g, Fiber 0g, Sodium: 1481mg, Potassium 239mg

176. Smoked Shrimp

Servings: 4   Cooking Time: 10 Minutes
Ingredients:
- 4 tablespoons olive oil
- 1 tablespoon Cajun seasoning
- 2 cloves garlic, minced
- 1 tablespoon lemon juice
- Salt to taste
- 2 lb. shrimp, peeled and deveined

Directions:
Combine all the ingredients in a sealable plastic bag. Toss to coat evenly.   Marinate in the refrigerator for 4 hours.   Set the wood pellet grill to high.   Preheat it for 15 minutes while the lid is closed.   Thread shrimp onto skewers.   Grill for 4 minutes per side.   Tips: Soak skewers first in water if you are using wooden skewers.

177. Grilled Shrimp Scampi

Servings: 4   Cooking Time: 10 Minutes
Ingredients:
- 1 lb raw shrimp, tail on
- 1/2 cup salted butter, melted
- 1/4 cup white wine, dry
- 1/2 tbsp fresh garlic, chopped
- 1 tbsp lemon juice
- 1/2 tbsp garlic powder
- 1/2 tbsp salt

Directions:
Preheat your wood pellet grill to 400°F with a cast iron inside.   In a mixing bowl, mix butter, wine, garlic, and juice then pour in the cast iron. Let the mixture mix for 4 minutes.   Sprinkle garlic and salt on the shrimp then place it on the cast iron. Grill for 10 minutes with the lid closed.   Remove the shrimp from the grill and serve when hot. Enjoy.

Nutrition Info: Calories 298, Total fat 24g, Saturated fat 15g, Total Carbs 2g, Net Carbs 2g, Protein 16g, Sugar 0g, Fiber 0g, Sodium: 1091mg, Potassium 389mg

178. Teriyaki Smoked Shrimp

Servings: 6   Cooking Time: 20 Minutes
Ingredients:
- Uncooked shrimp - 1 lb.
- Onion powder - ½ tbsp
- Garlic powder - ½ tbsp
- Teriyaki sauce - 4 tbsp
- Mayo - 4 tbsp
- Minced green onion - 2 tbsp
- Salt - ½ tbsp

Directions:
Remove the shells from the shrimp and wash thoroughly. Preheat the wood pellet grill to 450 degrees.   Season with garlic powder, onion powder, and salt.   Cook the shrimp for 5-6 minutes on each side.   Once cooked, remove the shrimp from the grill and garnish it with spring onion, teriyaki sauce, and mayo.

Nutrition Info: Carbohydrates: 2 g Protein: 16 g Sodium: 1241 mg Cholesterol: 190 mg

179. Charleston Crab Cakes With Remoulade

Servings: 4   Cooking Time: 45 Minutes
Ingredients:
- 1¼ cups mayonnaise
- ¼ cup yellow mustard
- 2 tablespoons sweet pickle relish, with its juices
- 1 tablespoon smoked paprika
- 2 teaspoons Cajun seasoning
- 2 teaspoons prepared horseradish
- 1 teaspoon hot sauce
- 1 garlic clove, finely minced
- 2 pounds fresh lump crabmeat, picked clean
- 20 butter crackers (such as Ritz brand), crushed
- 2 tablespoons Dijon mustard
- 1 cup mayonnaise
- 2 tablespoons freshly squeezed lemon juice
- 1 tablespoon salted butter, melted
- 1 tablespoon Worcestershire sauce
- 1 tablespoon Old Bay seasoning
- 2 teaspoons chopped fresh parsley
- 1 teaspoon ground mustard
- 2 eggs, beaten
- ¼ cup extra-virgin olive oil, divided

Directions:

For the remoulade: In a small bowl, combine the mayonnaise, mustard, pickle relish, paprika, Cajun seasoning, horseradish, hot sauce, and garlic. Refrigerate until ready to serve. For the crab cakes: Supply your smoker with wood pellets and follow the manufacturer's specific start-up procedure. Preheat, with the lid closed, to 375°F. Spread the crabmeat on a foil-lined baking sheet and place over indirect heat on the grill, with the lid closed, for 30 minutes. Remove from the heat and let cool for 15 minutes. While the crab cools, combine the crushed crackers, Dijon mustard, mayonnaise, lemon juice, melted butter, Worcestershire sauce, Old Bay, parsley, ground mustard, and eggs until well incorporated. Fold in the smoked crabmeat, then shape the mixture into 8 (1-inch-thick) crab cakes. In a large skillet or cast-iron pan on the grill, heat 2 tablespoons of olive oil. Add half of the crab cakes, close the lid, and smoke for 4 to 5 minutes on each side, or until crispy and golden brown. Remove the crab cakes from the pan and transfer to a wire rack to drain. Pat them to remove any excess oil. Repeat steps 6 and 7 with the remaining oil and crab cakes. Serve the crab cakes with the remoulade.

180. Togarashi Smoked Salmon

Servings: 10   Cooking Time: 20 Hours 15 Minutes
Ingredients:
- Salmon filet - 2 large
- Togarashi for seasoning
- For Brine:
- Brown sugar - 1 cup
- Water - 4 cups
- Kosher salt - ⅓ cup

Directions:
Remove all the thorns from the fish filet. Mix all the brine ingredients until the brown sugar is dissolved completely. Put the mix in a big bowl and add the filet to it. Leave the bowl to refrigerate for 16 hours. After 16 hours, remove the salmon from this mix. Wash and dry it. Place the salmon in the refrigerator for another 2-4 hours. (This step is important. DO NOT SKIP IT.) Season your salmon filet with Togarashi. Start the wood pellet grill with the 'smoke' option and place the salmon on it. Smoke for 4 hours. Make sure the temperature does not go above 180 degrees or below 130 degrees. Remove from the grill and serve it warm with a side dish of your choice.
Nutrition Info: Carbohydrates: 19 g Protein: 10 g Fat: 6 g Sodium: 3772 mg   Cholesterol: 29 mg

181. Citrus-smoked Trout

Servings: 6   Cooking Time: 1 To 2 Hours
Ingredients:
- 6 to 8 skin-on rainbow trout, cleaned and scaled
- 1 gallon orange juice
- ½ cup packed light brown sugar
- ¼ cup salt

- 1 tablespoon freshly ground black pepper
- Nonstick spray, oil, or butter, for greasing
- 1 tablespoon chopped fresh parsley
- 1 lemon, sliced

Directions:
Fillet the fish and pat dry with paper towels. Pour the orange juice into a large container with a lid and stir in the brown sugar, salt, and pepper. Place the trout in the brine, cover, and refrigerate for 1 hour. Cover the grill grate with heavy-duty aluminum foil. Poke holes in the foil and spray with cooking spray (see Tip). Supply your smoker with wood pellets and follow the manufacturer's specific start-up procedure. Preheat, with the lid closed, to 225°F. Remove the trout from the brine and pat dry. Arrange the fish on the foil-covered grill grate, close the lid, and smoke for 1 hour 30 minutes to 2 hours, or until flaky. Remove the fish from the heat. Serve garnished with the fresh parsley and lemon slices.

182. Cured Cold-smoked Lox

Servings: 6   Cooking Time: 6 Hours
Ingredients:
- ¼ cup salt
- ¼ cup sugar
- 1 tablespoon freshly ground black pepper
- 1 bunch dill, chopped
- 1 pound sashimi-grade salmon, skin removed
- 1 avocado, sliced
- 8 bagels
- 4 ounces cream cheese
- 1 bunch alfalfa sprouts
- 1 (5-ounce) jar capers

Directions:
In a small bowl, combine the salt, sugar, pepper, and fresh dill to make the curing mixture. Set aside. On a smooth surface, lay out a large piece of plastic wrap and spread half of the curing salt mixture in the middle, spreading it out to about the size of the salmon. Place the salmon on top of the curing salt. Top the fish with the remaining curing salt, covering it completely. Wrap the salmon, leaving the ends open to drain. Place the wrapped fish in a rimmed baking pan or dish lined with paper towels to soak up liquid. Place a weight on the salmon evenly, such as a pan with a couple of heavy jars of pickles on top. Put the salmon pan with weights in the refrigerator. Place something (a dishtowel, for example) under the back of the pan in order to slightly tip it down so the liquid drains away from the fish. Leave the salmon to cure in the refrigerator for 24 hours. Place the wood pellets in the smoker, but do not follow the start-up procedure and do not preheat. Remove the salmon from the refrigerator, unwrap it, rinse it off, and pat dry. Put the salmon in the smoker while still cold from the refrigerator to slow down the cooking process. You'll need to use a cold-smoker attachment or enlist the help of a smoker tube to hold the temperature at 80°F and maintain that for 6 hours to absorb smoke and complete the cold-smoking process. Remove the salmon from the smoker, place it in a sealed plastic bag,

and refrigerate for 24 hours. The salmon will be translucent all the way through. Thinly slice the lox and serve with sliced avocado, bagels, cream cheese, alfalfa sprouts, and capers.

183. Smoked Scallops

Servings: 6   Cooking Time: 15 Minutes
Ingredients:
- 2 pounds sea scallops
- 4 tbsp salted butter
- 2 tbsp lemon juice
- ½ tsp ground black pepper
- 1 garlic clove (minced)
- 1 kosher tsp salt
- 1 tsp freshly chopped tarragon

Directions:
Let the scallops dry using paper towels and drizzle all sides with salt and pepper to season   Place you're a cast iron pan in your grill and preheat the grill to 400°F with lid closed for 15 minutes.   Combine the butter and garlic in hot cast iron pan. Add the scallops and stir. Close grill lid and cook for 8 minutes. Flip the scallops and cook for an additional 7 minutes.   Remove the scallop from heat and let it rest for a few minutes.   Stir in the chopped tarragon. Serve and top with lemon juice.
Nutrition Info: Calories: 204 Cal Fat: 8.9 g
Carbohydrates: 4 g   Protein: 25.6 g Fiber: 0.1 g

184. Halibut With Garlic Pesto

Servings: 4   Cooking Time: 10 Minutes
Ingredients:
- 4 halibut fillets
- 1 cup olive oil
- Salt and pepper to taste
- 1/4 cup garlic, chopped
- 1/4 cup pine nuts

Directions:
Set the   wood pellet grill to smoke.   Establish fire for 5 minutes.   Set temperature to high.   Place a cast iron on a grill.   Season fish with salt and pepper. Add fish to the pan.   Drizzle with a little oil.   Sear for 4 minutes per side.   Prepare the garlic pesto by pulsing the remaining ingredients in the food processor until smooth.   Serve fish with garlic pesto.   Tips: You can also use other white fish fillets for this recipe.

185. Omega-3 Rich Salmon

Servings: 6   Cooking Time: 20 Minutes
Ingredients:
- 6 (6-oz.) skinless salmon fillets
- 1/3 C. olive oil
- ¼ C. spice rub
- ¼ C. honey
- 2 tbsp. Sriracha
- 2 tbsp. fresh lime juice

Directions:

Set the temperature of   Grill to 300 degrees F and preheat with closed lid for 15 minutes.   Coat salmon fillets with olive oil and season with rub evenly.   In a small bowl, mix together remaining ingredients. Arrange salmon fillets onto the grill, flat-side up and cook for about 7-10 minutes per side, coating with honey mixture once halfway through.   Serve hot alongside remaining honey mixture.
Nutrition Info: Calories per serving: 384;
Carbohydrates: 15.7g; Protein: 33g; Fat: 21.7g; Sugar: 11.6g; Sodium: 621mg; Fiber: 0g

186. Fish Fillets With Pesto

Servings: 6   Cooking Time: 15 Minutes
Ingredients:
- 2 cups fresh basil
- 1 cup parsley, chopped
- 1/2 cup walnuts
- 1/2 cup olive oil
- 1 cup Parmesan cheese, grated
- Salt and pepper to taste
- 4 white fish fillets

Directions:
Preheat the   wood pellet grill to high for 15 minutes while the lid is closed.   Add all the ingredients except fish to a food processor.   Pulse until smooth. Set aside. Season fish with salt and pepper.   Grill for 6 to 7 minutes per side.   Serve with the pesto sauce.   Tips: You can also spread a little bit of the pesto on the fish before grilling.

187. Buttered Crab Legs

Servings: 4   Cooking Time: 10 Minutes
Ingredients:
- 12 tablespoons butter
- 1 tablespoon parsley, chopped
- 1 tablespoon tarragon, chopped
- 1 tablespoon chives, chopped
- 1 tablespoon lemon juice
- 4 lb. king crab legs, split in the center

Directions:
Set the   wood pellet grill to 375 degrees F.   Preheat it for 15 minutes while lid is closed.   In a pan over medium heat, simmer the butter, herbs and lemon juice for 2 minutes.   Place the crab legs on the grill.   Pour half of the sauce on top.   Grill for 10 minutes.   Serve with the reserved butter sauce.   Tips: You can also use shrimp for this recipe.

188. Citrus Salmon

Servings: 6   Cooking Time: 30 Minutes
Ingredients:
- 2 (1-lb.) salmon fillets
- Salt and freshly ground black pepper, to taste
- 1 tbsp. seafood seasoning
- 2 lemons, sliced

- 2 limes, sliced

Directions:
Set the temperature of Grill to 225 degrees F and preheat with closed lid for 15 minutes. Season the salmon fillets with salt, black pepper and seafood seasoning evenly. Place the salmon fillets onto the grill and top each with lemon and lime slices evenly. Cook for about 30 minutes. Remove the salmon fillets from grill and serve hot.

Nutrition Info: Calories per serving: 327; Carbohydrates: 1g; Protein: 36.1g; Fat: 19.8g; Sugar: 0.2g; Sodium: 237mg; Fiber: 0.3g

189. Cod With Lemon Herb Butter

Servings: 4   Cooking Time: 15 Minutes
Ingredients:
- 4 tablespoons butter
- 1 clove garlic, minced
- 1 tablespoon tarragon, chopped
- 1 tablespoon lemon juice
- 1 teaspoon lemon zest
- Salt and pepper to taste
- 1 lb. cod fillet

Directions:
Preheat the wood pellet grill to high for 15 minutes while the lid is closed. In a bowl, mix the butter, garlic, tarragon, lemon juice and lemon zest, salt and pepper. Place the fish in a baking pan. Spread the butter mixture on top. Bake the fish for 15 minutes. Tips: You can also use other white fish fillet for this recipe.

190. Cajun Smoked Catfish

Servings: 4   Cooking Time: 2 Hours
Ingredients:
- 4 catfish fillets (5 ounces each)
- ½ cup Cajun seasoning
- 1 tsp ground black pepper
- 1 tbsp smoked paprika
- 1/4 tsp cayenne pepper
- 1 tsp hot sauce
- 1 tsp granulated garlic
- 1 tsp onion powder
- 1 tsp thyme
- 1 tsp salt or more to taste
- 2 tbsp chopped fresh parsley

Directions:
Pour water into the bottom of a square or rectangular dish. Add 4 tbsp salt. Arrange the catfish fillets into the dish. Cover the dish and refrigerate for 3 to 4 hours. Combine the paprika, cayenne, hot sauce, onion, salt, thyme, garlic, pepper and Cajun seasoning in a mixing bowl. Remove the fish from the dish and let it sit for a few minutes, or until it is at room temperature. Pat the fish fillets dry with a paper towel. Rub the seasoning mixture over each fillet generously. Start your grill on smoke, leaving the lid opened for 5 minutes, or until fire starts. Keep lid unopened and preheat to 200°F, using mesquite hardwood pellets. Arrange the fish fillets onto the grill grate and close the grill. Cook for about 2 hours, or until the fish is flaky. Remove the fillets from the grill and let the fillets rest for a few minutes to cool. Serve and garnish with chopped fresh parsley.

Nutrition Info: Calories: 204 Cal Fat: 11.1 g Carbohydrates: 2.7 g   Protein: 22.9 g Fiber: 0.6 g

POULTRY RECIPES

191. Smoked Whole Chicken

Servings: 6 To 8   Cooking Time: 4 Hours
Ingredients:
- 1 whole chicken
- 2 cups Tea Injectable (using Not-Just-for-Pork Rub)
- 2 tablespoons olive oil
- 1 batch Chicken Rub
- 2 tablespoons butter, melted

Directions:
Supply your smoker with wood pellets and follow the manufacturer's specific start-up procedure. Preheat the grill, with the lid closed, to 180°F.   Inject the chicken throughout with the tea injectable.   Coat the chicken all over with olive oil and season it with the rub. Using your hands, work the rub into the meat.   Place the chicken directly on the grill grate and smoke for 3 hours. Baste the chicken with the butter and increase the grill's temperature to 375°F. Continue to cook the chicken until its internal temperature reaches 170°F.   Remove the chicken from the grill and let it rest for 10 minutes, before carving and serving.

192. Hickory Smoked Chicken

Servings: 4   Cooking Time: 30 Minutes
Ingredients:
- 4 chicken breasts
- ¼ cup olive oil
- 1 teaspoon pressed garlic
- 1 tablespoon Worcestershire sauce
- Kirkland Sweet Mesquite Seasoning as needed
- 1 button   Honey Bourbon Sauce

Directions:
Place all ingredients in a bowl except for the Bourbon sauce. Massage the chicken until all parts are coated with the seasoning.   Allow to marinate in the fridge for 4 hours.   Once ready to cook, fire the   Grill to 350F. Use Hickory wood pellets and close the lid. Preheat for 15 minutes.   Place the chicken directly into the grill grate and cook for 30 minutes. Flip the chicken halfway through the cooking time.   Five minutes before the cooking time ends, brush all surfaces of the chicken with the Honey Bourbon Sauce.   Serve immediately.
Nutrition Info: Calories per serving: 622;
Protein: 60.5g; Carbs: 1.1g; Fat: 40.3g Sugar: 0.4g

193. Game Day Chicken Drumsticks

Servings: 8   Cooking Time: 1 Hour
Ingredients:
- For Brine:
- ½ C. brown sugar
- ½ C. kosher salt
- 5 C. water
- 2 (12-oz.) bottles beer
- 8 chicken drumsticks
- For Coating:
- ¼ C. olive oil
- ½ C. BBQ rub
- 1 tbsp. fresh parsley, minced
- 1 tbsp. fresh chives, minced
- ¾ C. BBQ sauce
- ¼ C. beer

Directions:
For brine: in a bucket, dissolve brown sugar and kosher salt in water and beer.   Place the chicken drumsticks in brine and refrigerate, covered for about 3 hours.   Set the temperature of   Grill to 275 degrees F and preheat with closed lid for 15 minutes.   Remove chicken drumsticks from brine and rinse under cold running water.   With paper towels, pat dry chicken drumsticks. Coat drumsticks with olive oil and rub with BBQ rub evenly.   Sprinkle the drumsticks with parsley and chives.   Arrange the chicken drumsticks onto the grill and cook for about 45 minutes.   Meanwhile, in a bowl, mix together BBQ sauce and beer.   Remove from grill and coat the drumsticks with BBQ sauce evenly.   Cook for about 15 minutes more.   Serve immediately.
Nutrition Info: Calories per serving: 448;
Carbohydrates: 20.5g; Protein: 47.2g; Fat: 16.1g; Sugar: 14.9g; Sodium: 9700mg; Fiber: 0.2g

194. Smoked And Fried Chicken Wings

Servings: 6   Cooking Time: 2 Hours
Ingredients:
- 3 pounds chicken wings
- 1 tbsp Goya adobo all-purpose seasoning
- Sauce of your choice

Directions:
Fire up your wood pellet grill and set it to smoke. Meanwhile, coat the chicken wings with adobo all-purpose seasoning. Place the chicken on the grill and smoke for 2 hours.   Remove the wings from the grill. Preheat oil to 375°F in a frying pan. Drop the wings in batches and let fry for 5 minutes or until the skin is crispy. Drain the oil and proceed with drizzling preferred sauce Drain oil and drizzle preferred sauce   Enjoy.
Nutrition Info: Calories: 755 Cal Fat: 55 g
Carbohydrates: 24 g   Protein: 39 g Fiber: 1 g

195. Cajun Chicken

Servings: 4   Cooking Time: 30 Minutes
Ingredients:
- 2 lb. chicken wings
- Poultry dry rub
- Cajun seasoning

Directions:
Season the chicken wings with the dry rub and Cajun seasoning.   Preheat the   to 350 degrees F for 15

minutes while the lid is closed.   Grill for 30 minutes, flipping twice.   Tips: You can also smoke the chicken before grilling.

196. Whole Smoked Chicken

Servings: 6   Cooking Time: 3 Hours
Ingredients:
- ½ cup salt
- 1 cup brown sugar
- 1 whole chicken (3 ½ pounds)
- 1 teaspoon minced garlic
- 1 lemon, halved
- 1 medium onion, quartered
- 3 whole cloves
- 5 sprigs of thyme

Directions:
Dissolve the salt and sugar in 4 liters of water. Once dissolved, place the chicken in the brine and allow to marinate for 24 hours.   When ready to cook, fire the Grill up to 250F and allow to preheat for 15 minutes with the lid closed. Use any wood pellet desired but we recommend using the maple wood pellet.   While the grill is preheating, remove the chicken from the brine and pat dry using paper towel. Rub the minced garlic all over the chicken. Stuff the cavity of the chicken with the remaining ingredients.   Tie the legs together with a natural string.   Place the stuffed chicken directly on the grill grate and smoke for 3 hours until the internal temperature of the chicken is 160F particularly in the breast part.   Take the chicken out and grill.
Nutrition Info: Calories per serving: 251;
Protein: 32.6g; Carbs: 19g; Fat: 4.3g Sugar: 17.3g

197. Wood Pellet Chile Lime Chicken

Servings: 1   Cooking Time: 15 Minutes
Ingredients:
- 1 chicken breast
- 1 tbsp oil
- 1 tbsp chile-lime seasoning

Directions:
Preheat your wood pellet to 400°F.   Brush the chicken breast with oil on all sides.   Sprinkle with seasoning and salt to taste.   Grill for 7 minutes per side or until the internal temperature reaches 165°F.   Serve when hot or cold and enjoy.
Nutrition Info: Calories: 131 Cal Fat: 5 g
Carbohydrates: 4 g   Protein: 19 g Fiber: 1 g

198. Special Occasion's Dinner Cornish Hen

Servings: 4   Cooking Time: 1 Hour
Ingredients:
- 4 Cornish game hens
- 4 fresh rosemary sprigs
- 4 tbsp. butter, melted
- 4 tsp. chicken rub

Directions:

Set the temperature of   Grill to 375 degrees F and preheat with closed lid for 15 minutes.   With paper towels, pat dry the hens.   Tuck the wings behind the backs and with kitchen strings, tie the legs together. Coat the outside of each hen with melted butter and sprinkle with rub evenly.   Stuff the cavity of each hen with a rosemary sprig.   Place the hens onto the grill and cook for about 50-60 minutes.   Remove the hens from grill and place onto a platter for about 10 minutes. Cut each hen into desired-sized pieces and serve.
Nutrition Info: Calories per serving: 430;
Carbohydrates: 2.1g; Protein: 25.4g; Fat: 33g; Sugar: 0g; Sodium: 331mg; Fiber: 0.7g

199. Chile-lime Rubbed Chicken

Servings: 6   Cooking Time: 40 Minutes
Ingredients:
- 3 tablespoons chili powder
- 2 tablespoons extra virgin olive oil
- 2 teaspoons lime zest
- 3 tablespoons lime juice
- 1 tablespoon garlic, minced
- 1 teaspoon ground coriander
- 1 teaspoon ground cumin
- 1 teaspoon dried oregano
- 1 ½ teaspoons salt
- 1 teaspoon ground black pepper
- A pinch of cinnamon
- 1 chicken, spatchcocked

Directions:
In a bowl, place the chili powder, olive oil, lime zest, juice, garlic, coriander, cumin, oregano, salt, pepper, cinnamon, and cinnamon in a bowl. Mix to form a paste. Place the chicken cut-side down on a chopping board and flatten using the heel of your hand. Carefully, break the breastbone to flatten the chicken.   Generously rub the spices all over the chicken and make sure to massage the chicken with the spice rub. Place in a baking dish and refrigerate for 24 hours in the fridge.   When ready to cook, fire the   Grill to 400F. Use maple wood pellets.   Close the grill lid and preheat for 15 minutes. Place the chicken breastbone-side down on the grill grate and cook for 40 minutes or until a thermometer inserted in the thickest part reads at 165F.   Make sure to flip the chicken halfway through the cooking time.   Once cooked, transfer to a plate and allow to rest before carving the chicken.
Nutrition Info: Calories per serving: 213;
Protein: 33.1g; Carbs: 3.8g; Fat: 7g Sugar: 0.5g

200. Grilled Sweet And Sour Chicken

Servings: 6   Cooking Time: 35 Minutes
Ingredients:
- 6 cups water
- 1/3 cup salt
- ¼ cup brown sugar
- ¼ cup soy sauce
- 6 chicken breasts, boneless

- 1 cup granulated white sugar
- ½ cup ketchup
- 1 cup apple cider vinegar
- 2 tablespoons soy sauce
- 1 teaspoon garlic powder

Directions:
Place the water, salt, brown sugar, and soy sauce in a large bowl. Stir until well combined. Add in the chicken breasts into the brine and allow to soak for 24 hours in the refrigerator.   Fire the   Grill to 350F. Use maple wood pellets. Close the grill lid and preheat for 15 minutes.   Place the breasts on the grill grate and cook for 35 minutes on each side with the lid closed. Flip the chicken halfway through the cooking time. Meanwhile, place the remaining ingredients in a bowl and stir until combined.   Ten minutes before the chicken breasts are cooked, brush with the sauce. Serve immediately.

Nutrition Info: Calories per serving: 675 ;
Protein: 61.9g; Carbs: 35.8g; Fat: 29.7g Sugar: 32.7g

201. Peppered Bbq Chicken Thighs

Servings: 6   Cooking Time: 35 Minutes
Ingredients:
- 6 bone-in chicken thighs
- Salt and pepper to taste
- Big Game Rub to taste, optional

Directions:
Place all ingredients in a bowl and allow to marinate in the fridge for at least 4 hours.   When ready to cook, fire the   Grill to 350F. Use apple wood pellet. Close the lid and preheat for 15 minutes.   Place the chicken directly on the grill grate and cook for 35 minutes. To check if the chicken is cooked thoroughly, insert a meat thermometer, and make sure that the internal temperature reads at 165F.   Serve the chicken immediately.

Nutrition Info: Calories per serving: 430;
Protein: 32g; Carbs: 1.2g; Fat: 32.1g; Sugar: 0.4g

202. Grilled Chicken

Servings: 6   Cooking Time: 1 Hour 10 Minutes;
Ingredients:
- 5 lb. whole chicken
- 1/2 cup oil
- chicken rub

Directions:
Preheat the   on the smoke setting with the lid open for 5 minutes. Close the lid and let it heat for 15 minutes or until it reaches 450..   Use bakers twine to tie the chicken legs together then rub it with oil. Coat the chicken with the rub and place it on the grill.   Grill for 70 minutes with the lid closed or until it reaches an internal temperature of 165F.   Remove the chicken from the   and let rest for 15 minutes. Cut and serve.

Nutrition Info: Calories 935, Total fat 53g, Saturated fat 15g, Total carbs 0g, Net carbs 0g Protein 107g, Sugars 0g, Fiber 0g, Sodium 320mg

203. Smoked Chicken And Potatoes

Servings: 4   Cooking Time: 1 Hour And 30 Minutes
Ingredients:
- 1 2.5-pounds rotisserie chicken
- 2 tablespoon coconut sugar
- 1 tablespoons onion powder
- 2 tablespoon garlic powder
- 1 teaspoon cayenne pepper powder
- 2 teaspoon kosher salt
- 4 tablespoons olive oil
- 2 pounds creamer potatoes, scrubbed and halved
- A dash of black pepper powder

Directions:
Place the chicken in a bowl. In a smaller bowl, combine the coconut sugar, onion powder, garlic powder, cayenne pepper powder, and salt. Add in the olive oil. Rub the mixture into the chicken and allow to marinate for 4 hours in the fridge.   Fire the   Grill to 400F and close the lid. Preheat to 15 minutes.   Place the seasoned chicken in a heat-proof dish and place the potatoes around the chicken. Season the potatoes with salt. Place in the grill and cook for 30 minutes. Lower the heat to 250F and cook for another hour.   Insert a meat thermometer in the thickest part of the chicken and make sure that the temperature reads at 165F. Flip the chicken halfway through the cooking time for even browning.

Nutrition Info: Calories per serving: 991;
Protein: 79.7g; Carbs: 49.8g; Fat: 73.6g Sugar: 6.5g

204. Crispy & Juicy Chicken

Servings: 6   Cooking Time: 5 Hours
Ingredients:
- ¾ C. dark brown sugar
- ½ C. ground espresso beans
- 1 tbsp. ground cumin
- 1 tbsp. ground cinnamon
- 1 tbsp. garlic powder
- 1 tbsp. cayenne pepper
- Salt and freshly ground black pepper, to taste
- 1 (4-lb.) whole chicken, neck and giblets removed

Directions:
Set the temperature of   Grill to 200-225 degrees F and preheat with closed lid for 15 minutes.   In a bowl, mix together brown sugar, ground espresso, spices, salt and black pepper.   Rub the chicken with spice mixture generously.   Place the chicken onto the grill and cook for about 3-5 hours.   Remove chicken from grill and place onto a cutting board for about 10 minutes before carving.   With a sharp knife, cut the chicken into desired-sized pieces and serve.

Nutrition Info: Calories per serving: 540;
Carbohydrates: 20.7g; Protein: 88.3g; Fat: 9.6g; Sugar: 18.1g; Sodium: 226mg; Fiber: 1.2g

205. Smoked Fried Chicken

Servings: 6   Cooking Time: 3 Hours

Ingredients:
- 3.5 lb. chicken
- Vegetable oil
- Salt and pepper to taste
- 2 tablespoons hot sauce
- 1 quart buttermilk
- 2 tablespoons brown sugar
- 1 tablespoon poultry dry rub
- 2 tablespoons onion powder
- 2 tablespoons garlic powder
- 2 1/2 cups all-purpose flour
- Peanut oil

Directions:
Set the wood pellet grill to 200 degrees F. Preheat it for 15 minutes while the lid is closed. Drizzle chicken with vegetable oil and sprinkle with salt and pepper. Smoke chicken for 2 hours and 30 minutes. In a bowl, mix the hot sauce, buttermilk and sugar. Soak the smoked chicken in the mixture. Cover and refrigerate for 1 hour. In another bowl, mix the dry rub, onion powder, garlic powder and flour. Coat the chicken with the mixture. Heat the peanut oil in a pan over medium heat. Fry the chicken until golden and crispy. Tips: Drain chicken on paper towels before serving.

206. Grilled Buffalo Chicken

Servings: 6   Cooking Time: 20 Minutes
Ingredients:
- 5 chicken breasts, boneless and skinless
- 2 tbsp homemade BBQ rub
- 1 cup homemade Cholula Buffalo sauce

Directions:
Preheat the to 400F. Slice the chicken breast lengthwise into strips. Season the slices with BBQ rub. Place the chicken slices on the grill and paint both sides with buffalo sauce. Cook for 4 minutes with the lid closed. Flip the breasts, paint again with sauce and cook until the internal temperature reaches 165F. Remove the chicken from the and serve when warm.
Nutrition Info: Calories 176, Total fat 4g, Saturated fat 1g, Total carbs 1g, Net carbs 1g Protein 32g, Sugars 1g, Fiber 0g, Sodium 631mg

207. Turkey Meatballs

Servings: 8   Cooking Time: 40 Minutes
Ingredients:
- 1 1/4 lb. ground turkey
- 1/2 cup breadcrumbs
- 1 egg, beaten
- 1/4 cup milk
- 1 teaspoon onion powder
- 1/4 cup Worcestershire sauce
- Pinch garlic salt
- Salt and pepper to taste
- 1 cup cranberry jam
- 1/2 cup orange marmalade
- 1/2 cup chicken broth

Directions:
In a large bowl, mix the ground turkey, breadcrumbs, egg, milk, onion powder, Worcestershire sauce, garlic salt, salt and pepper. Form meatballs from the mixture. Preheat the wood pellet grill to 350 degrees F for 15 minutes while the lid is closed. Add the turkey meatballs to a baking pan. Place the baking pan on the grill. Cook for 20 minutes. In a pan over medium heat, simmer the rest of the ingredients for 10 minutes. Add the grilled meatballs to the pan. Coat with the mixture. Cook for 10 minutes. Tips: You can add chili powder to the meatball mixture if you want spicy flavor.

208. Cornish Game Hen

Servings: 4   Cooking Time: 2 To 3 Hours
Ingredients:
- 4 Cornish game hens
- Extra-virgin olive oil, for rubbing
- 2 teaspoons salt
- 1 teaspoon freshly ground black pepper
- 1 teaspoon celery seeds

Directions:
Supply your smoker with wood pellets and follow the manufacturer's specific start-up procedure. Preheat, with the lid closed, to 275°F. Rub the game hens over and under the skin with olive oil and season all over with the salt, pepper, and celery seeds. Place the birds directly on the grill grate, close the lid, and smoke for 2 to 3 hours, or until a meat thermometer inserted in each bird reads 170°F. Serve the Cornish game hens hot.

209. Smoked Whole Duck

Servings: 6   Cooking Time: 2 Hours 30 Minutes
Ingredients:
- 5 pounds whole duck (trimmed of any excess fat)
- 1 small onion (quartered)
- 1 apple (wedged)
- 1 orange (quartered)
- 1 tbsp freshly chopped parsley
- 1 tbsp freshly chopped sage
- ½ tsp onion powder
- 2 tsp smoked paprika
- 1 tsp dried Italian seasoning
- 1 tbsp dried Greek seasoning
- 1 tsp pepper or to taste
- 1 tsp sea salt or to taste

Directions:
Remove giblets and rinse duck, inside and pour, under cold running water. Pat dry with paper towels. Use the tip of a sharp knife to cut the duck skin all over. Be careful not to cut through the meat. Tie the duck legs together with butcher's string. To make a rub, combine the onion powder, pepper, salt, Italian seasoning, Greek seasoning, and paprika in a mixing bowl. Insert the orange, onion, and apple to the duck cavity. Stuff the duck with freshly chopped parsley and sage. Season all sides of the duck generously with rub mixture. Start your pellet grill on smoke mode,

leaving the lip open or until the fire starts. Close the lid and preheat the grill to 325°F for 10 minutes. Place the duck on the grill grate. Roast for 2 to 2½ hours, or until the duck skin is brown and the internal temperature of the thigh reaches 160°F. Remove the duck from heat and let it rest for a few minutes. Cut into sizes and serve.

Nutrition Info: Calories: 809 Total Fat: 42.9 g Saturated Fat: 15.8 g Cholesterol: 337 mg Sodium: 638 mg Total Carbohydrate: 11.7 g Dietary Fiber: 2.4 g Total Sugars: 7.5 g Protein: 89.6 g

210. Perfectly Smoked Turkey Legs

Servings: 6   Cooking Time: 4 Hours
Ingredients:
- For Turkey:
- 3 tbsp. Worcestershire sauce
- 1 tbsp. canola oil
- 6 turkey legs
- For Rub:
- ¼ C. chipotle seasoning
- 1 tbsp. brown sugar
- 1 tbsp. paprika
- For Sauce:
- 1 C. white vinegar
- 1 tbsp. canola oil
- 1 tbsp. chipotle BBQ sauce

Directions:
For turkey in a bowl, add the Worcestershire sauce and canola oil and mix well. With your fingers, loosen the skin of legs. With your fingers coat the legs under the skin with oil mixture. In another bowl, mix together rub ingredients. Rub the spice mixture under and outer surface of turkey legs generously. Transfer the legs into a large sealable bag and refrigerate for about 2-4 hours. Remove the turkey legs from refrigerator and set aside at room temperature for at least 30 minutes before cooking. Set the temperature of Grill to 200-220 degrees F and preheat with closed lid for 15 minutes. In a small pan, mix together all sauce ingredients on low heat and cook until warmed completely, stirring continuously. Place the turkey legs onto the grill cook for about 3½-4 hours, coating with sauce after every 45 minutes. Serve hot.

Nutrition Info: Calories per serving: 430; Carbohydrates: 4.9g; Protein: 51.2g; Fat: 19.5g; Sugar: 3.9g; Sodium: 1474mg; Fiber: 0.5g

211. Barbecue Chicken Wings

Servings: 4   Cooking Time: 15 Minutes
Ingredients:
- Fresh chicken wings
- Salt to taste
- Pepper to taste
- Garlic powder
- Onion powder
- Cayenne
- Paprika

- Seasoning salt
- Bbq sauce to taste

Directions:
Preheat the wood pellet grill to low. In a mixing bowl, mix all the seasoning ingredients then toss the chicken wings until well coated. Place the wings on the grill and cook for 20 minutes or until the wings are fully cooked. Let rest to cool for 5 minutes then toss with bbq sauce. Serve with orzo and salad. Enjoy.

Nutrition Info: Calories 311, Total fat 22g, Saturated fat 4g, Total carbs 22g, Net carbs 19g, Protein 22g, Sugar 12g, Fiber 3g, Sodium: 1400mg

212. Grill Bbq Chicken Breasts

Servings: 4   Cooking Time: 30 Minutes
Ingredients:
- 4 whole chicken breasts, deboned
- ¼ cup olive oil
- 1 teaspoon pressed garlic
- 1 teaspoon Worcestershire sauce
- 1 teaspoon cayenne pepper powder
- ½ cup 'Que BBQ Sauce

Directions:
In a bowl, combine all ingredients except for the 'Que BBQ Sauce and make sure to rub the chicken breasts until coated with the mixture. Allow to marinate in the fridge for at least overnight. Place the preferred wood pellets into the Grill and fire the grill. Allow temperature to rise to 500F and preheat for 5 minutes. Reduce the temperature to 165F. Place the chicken on the grill grate and cook for 30 minutes. Five minutes before the chicken is done, glaze the chicken with 's BBQ sauce. Serve immediately.

Nutrition Info: Calories per serving: 631; Protein: 61g; Carbs: 2.9g; Fat: 40.5g Sugar: 1.5g

213. Rustic Maple Smoked Chicken Wings

Servings: 16   Cooking Time: 35 Minutes
Ingredients:
- 16 chicken wings
- 1 tablespoon olive oil
- 1 tablespoon Chicken Rub
- 1 cup 'Que BBQ Sauce or other commercial BBQ sauce of choice

Directions:
Place all ingredients in a bowl except for the BBQ sauce. Massage the chicken breasts so that it is coated with the marinade. Place in the fridge to marinate for at least 4 hours. Fire the Grill to 350F. Use maple wood pellets. Close the grill lid and preheat for 15 minutes. Place the wings on the grill grate and cook for 12 minutes on each side with the lid closed. Once the chicken wings are done, place in a clean bowl. Pour over the BBQ sauce and toss to coat with the sauce.

Nutrition Info: Calories per serving: 230 ; Protein: 37.5g; Carbs: 2.2g; Fat: 7g Sugar: 1.3g

214. Chicken Breast

Servings: 6   Cooking Time: 15 Minutes
Ingredients:
- 3 chicken breasts
- 1 tbsp avocado oil
- 1/4 tbsp garlic powder
- 1/4 tbsp onion powder
- 3/4 tbsp salt
- 1/4 tbsp pepper

Directions:
Preheat your   to 375F   Cut the chicken breast into halves lengthwise then coat with avocado oil.   Season with garlic powder, onion powder, salt, and pepper. Place the chicken on the grill and cook for 7 minutes on each side or until the internal temperature reaches 165F
Nutrition Info: Calories 120, Total fat 4g, Saturated fat 1g, Total carbs 0g, Net carbs 0g Protein 19g, Sugars 0g, Fiber 0g, Sodium 309mg

215. South-east-asian Chicken Drumsticks

Servings: 6   Cooking Time: 2 Hours
Ingredients:
- 1 C. fresh orange juice
- ¼ C. honey
- 2 tbsp. sweet chili sauce
- 2 tbsp. hoisin sauce
- 2 tbsp. fresh ginger, grated finely
- 2 tbsp. garlic, minced
- 1 tsp. Sriracha
- ½ tsp. sesame oil
- 6 chicken drumsticks

Directions:
Set the temperature of   Grill to 225 degrees F and preheat with closed lid for 15 minutes, using charcoal. In a bowl, place all ingredients except for chicken drumsticks and mix until well combined.   Reserve half of honey mixture in a small bowl.   In the bowl of remaining sauce, add drumsticks and mix well. Arrange the chicken drumsticks onto the grill and cook for about 2 hours, basting with remaining sauce occasionally.   Serve hot.
Nutrition Info: Calories per serving: 385;
Carbohydrates: 22.7g; Protein: 47.6g; Fat: 10.5g; Sugar: 18.6g; Sodium: 270mg; Fiber: 0.6g

216. Asian Miso Chicken Wings

Servings: 6   Cooking Time: 25 Minutes
Ingredients:
- 2 lb chicken wings
- 3/4 cup soy
- 1/2 cup pineapple juice
- 1 tbsp sriracha
- 1/8 cup miso
- 1/8 cup gochujang
- 1/2 cup water
- 1/2 cup oil
- Togarashi

Directions:
Preheat the   to 375F   Combine all the ingredients except togarashi in a zip lock bag. Toss until the chicken wings are well coated. Refrigerate for 12 hours   Pace the wings on the grill grates and close the lid. Cook for 25 minutes or until the internal temperature reaches 165F Remove the wings from the   and sprinkle Togarashi. Serve when hot and enjoy.
Nutrition Info: Calories 703, Total fat 56g, Saturated fat 14g, Total carbs 24g, Net carbs 23g Protein 27g, Sugars 6g, Fiber 1g, Sodium 1156mg

217. Chicken Cordon Bleu

Servings: 6   Cooking Time: 40 Minutes
Ingredients:
- 6 boneless skinless chicken breasts
- 6 slices of ham
- 12 slices swiss cheese
- 1cup panko breadcrumbs
- ½ cup all-purpose flour
- 1tsp ground black pepper or to taste
- 1tsp salt or to taste
- 4tbsp grated parmesan cheese
- 2tbsp melted butter
- ½ tsp garlic powder
- ½ tsp thyme
- ¼ tsp parsley

Directions:
Butterfly the chicken breast with a pairing knife. Place the chicken breast in between 2 plastic wraps and pound with a mallet until the chicken breasts are ¼ inch thick. Place a plastic wrap on a flat surface. Place one fat chicken breast on it.   Place one slice of swiss cheese on the chicken. Place one slice of ham over the cheese and place another cheese slice over the ham.   Roll the chicken breast tightly. Fold both ends of the roll tightly. Pin both ends of the rolled chicken breast with a toothpick.   Repeat step 3 and 4 for the remaining chicken breasts   In a mixing bowl, combine the all-purpose flour, ½ tsp salt, and ½ tsp pepper. Set aside. In another mixing bowl, combine breadcrumbs, parmesan, butter, garlic, thyme, parsley, ½ tsp salt, and ½ tsp pepper. Set aside.   Break the eggs into another mixing bowl and whisk. Set aside.   Grease a baking sheet.   Bake one chicken breast roll. Dip into the flour mixture, brush with eggs and dip into breadcrumb mixture. The chicken breast should be coated.   Place it on the baking sheet.   Repeat steps 9 and 10 for the remaining breast rolls.   Preheat your grill to 375°F with the lid closed for 15 minutes.   Place the baking sheet on the grill and cook for about 40 minutes, or until the chicken is golden brown.   Remove the baking sheet from the grill and let the chicken rest for a few minutes.   Slice cordon bleu and serve.
Nutrition Info: Calories: 560 Total Fat: 27.4 g Saturated Fat: 15.9 g Cholesterol: 156mg Sodium: 1158 mg Total Carbohydrate: 23.2 g Dietary Fiber: 1.1 g Total Sugars: 1.2 g Protein: 54.3 g

218. Maple Turkey Breast

Servings: 4   Cooking Time: 2 Hours
Ingredients:
- 3 tablespoons olive oil
- 3 tablespoons dark brown sugar
- 3 tablespoons garlic, minced
- 2 tablespoons Cajun seasoning
- 2 tablespoons Worcestershire sauce
- 6 lb. turkey breast fillets

Directions:
Combine olive oil, sugar, garlic, Cajun seasoning and Worcestershire sauce in a bowl.   Soak the turkey breast fillets in the marinade.   Cover and marinate for 4 hours.   Grill the turkey at 180 degrees F for 2 hours. Tips: You can also sprinkle dry rub on the turkey before grilling.

219. Easy Rapid-fire Roast Chicken

Servings: 4   Cooking Time: 1 To 2 Hours
Ingredients:
- 1 (4-pound) whole chicken, giblets removed
- Extra-virgin olive oil, for rubbing
- 3 tablespoons Greek seasoning
- Juice of 1 lemon
- Butcher's string

Directions:
Supply your smoker with wood pellets and follow the manufacturer's specific start-up procedure. Preheat, with the lid closed, to 450°F.   Rub the bird generously all over with oil, including inside the cavity.   Sprinkle the Greek seasoning all over and under the skin of the bird, and squeeze the lemon juice over the breast. Tuck the chicken wings behind the back and tie the legs together with butcher's string or cooking twine.   Put the chicken directly on the grill, breast-side up, close the lid, and roast for 1 hour to 1 hour 30 minutes, or until a meat thermometer inserted in the thigh reads 165°F. Let the meat rest for 10 minutes before carving.

220. Chicken Fajitas On A Wood Pellet Grill

Servings: 10   Cooking Time: 20 Minutes
Ingredients:
- Chicken breast - 2 lbs, thin sliced
- Red bell pepper - 1 large
- Onion - 1 large
- Orange bell pepper - 1 large
- Seasoning mix
- Oil - 2 tbsp
- Onion powder - ½ tbsp
- Granulated garlic - ½ tbsp
- Salt - 1 tbsp

Directions:
Preheat the grill to 450 degrees.   Mix the seasonings and oil.   Add the chicken slices to the mix.   Line a large pan with a non-stick baking sheet.   Let the pan heat for 10 minutes.   Place the chicken, peppers, and other vegetables in the grill.   Grill for 10 minutes or until the chicken is cooked.   Remove it from the grill and serve with warm tortillas and vegetables.
Nutrition Info: Carbohydrates: 5 g Protein: 29 g Fat: 6 g Sodium: 360 mg Cholesterol: 77 mg

221. Chicken Wings

Servings: 4   Cooking Time: 15 Minutes
Ingredients:
- Fresh chicken wings
- Salt to taste
- Pepper to taste
- Garlic powder
- Onion powder
- Cayenne
- Paprika
- Seasoning salt
- Barbeque sauce to taste

Directions:
Preheat the wood pellet grill to low. Mix seasoning and coat on chicken. Put the wings on the grill and cook. Place the wings on the grill and cook for 20 minutes or until the wings are fully cooked. Let rest to cool for 5 minutes then toss with barbeque sauce. Serve with orzo and salad. Enjoy.
Nutrition Info: Calories: 311 Cal Fat: 22 g Carbohydrates: 22 g   Protein: 22 g Fiber: 3 g

222. Beer Can–smoked Chicken

Servings: 3 To 4   Cooking Time: 3 To 4 Hours
Ingredients:
- 8 tablespoons (1 stick) unsalted butter, melted
- ½ cup apple cider vinegar
- ½ cup Cajun seasoning, divided
- 1 teaspoon garlic powder
- 1 teaspoon onion powder
- 1 (4-pound) whole chicken, giblets removed
- Extra-virgin olive oil, for rubbing
- 1 (12-ounce) can beer
- 1 cup apple juice
- ½ cup extra-virgin olive oil

Directions:
In a small bowl, whisk together the butter, vinegar, ¼ cup of Cajun seasoning, garlic powder, and onion powder.   Use a meat-injecting syringe to inject the liquid into various spots in the chicken. Inject about half of the mixture into the breasts and the other half throughout the rest of the chicken.   Rub the chicken all over with olive oil and apply the remaining ¼ cup of Cajun seasoning, being sure to rub under the skin as well. Drink or discard half the beer and place the opened beer can on a stable surface.   Place the bird's cavity on top of the can and position the chicken so it will sit up by itself. Prop the legs forward to make the bird more stable, or buy an inexpensive, specially made stand to hold the beer can and chicken in place.   Supply your smoker with wood pellets and follow the manufacturer's specific start-up procedure. Preheat, with the lid closed, to 250°F. In a clean 12-ounce spray bottle, combine the apple juice

and olive oil. Cover and shake the mop sauce well before each use.   Carefully put the chicken on the grill. Close the lid and smoke the chicken for 3 to 4 hours, spraying with the mop sauce every hour, until golden brown and a meat thermometer inserted in the thickest part of the thigh reads 165°F. Keep a piece of aluminum foil handy to loosely cover the chicken if the skin begins to brown too quickly.   Let the meat rest for 5 minutes before carving.

223. Authentic Holiday Turkey Breast

Servings: 6   Cooking Time: 4 Hours
Ingredients:
- ½ C. honey
- ¼ C. dry sherry
- 1 tbsp. butter
- 2 tbsp. fresh lemon juice
- Salt, to taste
- 1 (3-3½-pound) skinless, boneless turkey breast

Directions:
In a small pan, place honey, sherry and butter over low heat and cook until the mixture becomes smooth, stirring continuously.   Remove from heat and stir in lemon juice and salt. Set aside to cool.   Transfer the honey mixture and turkey breast in a sealable bag. Seal the bag and shake to coat well.   Refrigerate for about 6-10 hours.   Set the temperature of Grill to 225-250 degrees F and preheat with closed lid for 15 minutes.   Place the turkey breast onto the grill and cook for about 2½-4 hours or until desired doneness. Remove turkey breast from grill and place onto a cutting board for about 15-20 minutes before slicing.   With a sharp knife, cut the turkey breast into desired-sized slices and serve.

Nutrition Info: Calories per serving: 443; Carbohydrates: 23.7g; Protein: 59.2g; Fat: 11.4g; Sugar: 23.4g; Sodium: 138mg; Fiber: 0.1g

224. Chile Lime Chicken

Servings: 1   Cooking Time: 15 Minutes
Ingredients:
- 1 chicken breast
- 1 tbsp oil
- 1 tbsp spiceology Chile Lime Seasoning

Directions:
Preheat your   to 400F.   Brush the chicken breast with oil then sprinkle the chile-lime seasoning and salt. Place the chicken breast on the grill and cook for 7 minutes on each side or until the internal temperature reaches 165F.   Serve when hot and enjoy.
Nutrition Info: Calories 131, Total fat 5g, Saturated fat 1g, Total carbs 4g, Net carbs 3g Protein 19g, Sugars 1g, Fiber 1g, Sodium 235mg

225. Wood Pellet Smoked Cornish Hens

Servings: 6   Cooking Time: 1 Hour

Ingredients:
- 6 Cornish hens
- 3 tbsp avocado oil
- 6 tbsp rub of choice

Directions:
Fire up the wood pellet and preheat it to 275°F.   Rub the hens with oil then coat generously with rub. Place the hens on the grill with the chest breast side down. Smoke for 30 minutes. Flip the hens and increase the grill temperature to 400°F. Cook until the internal temperature reaches 165°F.   Remove from the grill and let rest for 10 minutes before serving. Enjoy.
Nutrition Info: Calories: 696 Cal Fat: 50 g Carbohydrates: 1 g   Protein: 57 g Fiber: 0 g

226. Wild Turkey Egg Rolls

Servings: 4-6   Cooking Time: 40 Minutes
Ingredients:
- Corn - ½ cup
- Leftover wild turkey meat - 2 cups
- Black beans - ½ cup
- Taco seasoning - 3 tbsp
- Water ½ cup
- Rotel chilies and tomatoes - 1 can
- Egg roll wrappers- 12
- Cloves of minced garlic- 4
- 1 chopped Poblano pepper or 2 jalapeno peppers
- Chopped white onion - ½ cup

Directions:
Add some olive oil to a fairly large skillet. Heat it over medium heat on a stove.   Add peppers and onions. Sauté the mixture for 2-3 minutes until it turns soft. Add some garlic and sauté for another 30 seconds. Add the Rotel chilies and beans to the mixture. Keeping mixing the content gently. Reduce the heat and then simmer.   After about 4-5 minutes, pour in the taco seasoning and ⅓ cup of water over the meat. Mix everything and coat the meat thoroughly. If you feel that it is a bit dry, you can add 2 tbsp of water. Keep cooking until everything is heated all the way through. Remove the content from the heat and box it to store in a refrigerator. Before you stuff the mixture into the egg wrappers, it should be completely cool to avoid breaking the rolls.   Place a spoonful of the cooked mixture in each wrapper and then wrap it securely and tightly. Do the same with all the wrappers.   Preheat the pellet grill and brush it with some oil. Cook the egg rolls for 15 minutes on both sides until the exterior is nice and crispy. Remove them from the grill and enjoy with your favorite salsa!
Nutrition Info: Carbohydrates: 26.1 g Protein: 9.2 g Fat: 4.2 g Sodium: 373.4 mg   Cholesterol: 19.8 mg

227. Lemon Chicken Breast

Servings: 4   Cooking Time: 30 Minutes
Ingredients:
- 6 chicken breasts, skinless and boneless
- ½ cup oil

- 1-3 fresh thyme sprigs
- 1teaspoon ground black pepper
- 2teaspoon salt
- 2teaspoons honey
- 1garlic clove, chopped
- 1lemon, juiced and zested
- Lemon wedges

Directions:
Take a bowl and prepare the marinade by mixing thyme, pepper, salt, honey, garlic, lemon zest, and juice. Mix well until dissolved   Add oil and whisk   Clean breasts and pat them dry, place in a bag alongside marinade and let them sit in the fridge for 4 hours   Preheat your smoker to 400 degrees F   Drain chicken and smoke until the internal temperature reaches 165 degrees, for about 15 minutes   Serve and enjoy!
Nutrition Info: Calories: 230 Fats: 7g Carbs: 1g Fiber: 2g

228. Cinco De Mayo Chicken Enchiladas

Servings: 6   Cooking Time: 45 Minutes
Ingredients:
- 6 cups diced cooked chicken
- 3 cups grated Monterey Jack cheese, divided
- 1 cup sour cream
- 1 (4-ounce) can chopped green chiles
- 2 (10-ounce) cans red or green enchilada sauce, divided
- 12 (8-inch) flour tortillas
- ½ cup chopped scallions
- ¼ cup chopped fresh cilantro

Directions:
Supply your smoker with wood pellets and follow the manufacturer's specific start-up procedure. Preheat, with the lid closed, to 350°F.   In a large bowl, combine the cooked chicken, 2 cups of cheese, the sour cream, and green chiles to make the filling.   Pour one can of enchilada sauce in the bottom of a 9-by-13-inch baking dish or aluminum pan.   Spoon ⅓ cup of the filling on each tortilla and roll up securely.   Transfer the tortillas seam-side down to the baking dish, then pour the remaining can of enchilada sauce over them, coating all exposed surfaces of the tortillas.   Sprinkle the remaining 1 cup of cheese over the enchiladas and cover tightly with aluminum foil.   Bake on the grill, with the lid closed, for 30 minutes, then remove the foil. Continue baking with the lid closed for 15 minutes, or until bubbly.   Garnish the enchiladas with the chopped scallions and cilantro and serve immediately.

229. Wood Pellet Grilled Buffalo Chicken Leg

Servings: 6   Cooking Time: 25 Minutes
Ingredients:
- 12 chicken legs
- 1/2 tbsp salt
- 1 tbsp buffalo seasoning

- 1 cup buffalo sauce

Directions:
Preheat your wood pellet grill to 325°F.   Toss the legs in salt and buffalo seasoning then place them on the preheated grill.   Grill for 40 minutes ensuring you turn them twice through the cooking.   Brush the legs with buffalo sauce and cook for an additional 10 minutes or until the internal temperature reaches 165°F.   Remove the legs from the grill, brush with more sauce, and serve when hot.
Nutrition Info: Calories: 956 Cal Fat: 47 g Carbohydrates: 1 g   Protein: 124 g Fiber: 0 g

230. Hickory Smoked Chicken Leg And Thigh Quarters

Servings: 6   Cooking Time: 2 Hours
Ingredients:
- 6 chicken legs (with thigh and drumsticks)
- 2 tablespoons olive oil
- Poultry Rub to taste

Directions:
Place all ingredients in a bowl and mix until the chicken pieces are coated in oil and rub. Allow to marinate for at least 2 hours.   Fire the   Grill to 180F. Close the lid and allow to preheat for 10 minutes. Use hickory wood pellets to smoke your chicken.   Arrange the chicken on the grill grate and smoke for one hour. Increase the temperature to 350F and continue cooking for another hour until the chicken is golden and the juices run clean.   To check if the meat is cooked, insert a meat thermometer, and   make sure that the temperature on the thickest part of the chicken registers at 165F.   Remove the chicken and serve.
Nutrition Info: Calories per serving: 358 ;
Protein: 50.8g; Carbs: 0g; Fat: 15.7g Sugar:0 g

231. Smoked Cornish Hens

Servings: 6   Cooking Time: 1 Hour
Ingredients:
- 6 Cornish hens
- 3 tbsp canola oil
- 6 tbsp rub

Directions:
Preheat your   to 275F.   Meanwhile, rub the hens with canola oil then with your favorite rub.   Place the hens on the grill with the breast side down. Smoke for 30 minutes.   Flip the hens and increase the temperature to 400F. Cook until the internal temperature reaches 165F.   Remove the hens from the grill and let rest for 10 minutes before serving.
Nutrition Info: Calories 696, Total fat 50g, Saturated fat 13g, Total carbs 1g, Net carbs 1g Protein 57g, Sugars 0g, Fiber 0g, Sodium 165mg

232. Hot And Sweet Spatchcocked Chicken

Servings: 8   Cooking Time: 55 Minutes

Ingredients:
- 1 whole chicken, spatchcocked
- ¼ cup   Chicken Rub
- 2 tablespoons olive oil
- ½ cup   Sweet and Heat BBQ Sauce

Directions:
Place the chicken breastbone-side down on a flat surface and press the breastbone to break it and flatten the chicken. Sprinkle the   Chicken Rub all over the chicken and massage until the bird is seasoned well. Allow the chicken to rest in the fridge for at least 12 hours.   When ready to cook, fire the   Grill to 350F. Use preferred wood pellets. Close the grill lid and preheat for 15 minutes.   Before cooking the chicken, baste with oil. Place on the grill grate and cook on both sides for 55 minutes.   20 minutes before the cooking time, baste the chicken with   Sweet and Heat BBQ Sauce. Continue cooking until a meat thermometer inserted in the thickest part of the chicken reads at 165F.   Allow to rest before carving the chicken.

Nutrition Info: Calories per serving: 200; Protein: 30.6g; Carbs: 1.1g; Fat: 7.4g Sugar: 0.6g

233. Buffalo Wings

Servings: 2 To 3   Cooking Time: 35 Minutes
Ingredients:
- 1 pound chicken wings
- 1 batch Chicken Rub
- 1 cup Frank's Red-Hot Sauce, Buffalo wing sauce, or similar

Directions:
Supply your smoker with wood pellets and follow the manufacturer's specific start-up procedure. Preheat the grill, with the lid closed, to 300°F.   Season the chicken wings with the rub. Using your hands, work the rub into the meat.   Place the wings directly on the grill grate and smoke until their internal temperature reaches 160°F.   Baste the wings with the sauce and continue to smoke until the wings' internal temperature reaches 170°F.

234. Smoked Turkey Wings

Servings: 2   Cooking Time: 1 Hour
Ingredients:
- 4 turkey wings
- 1 batch Sweet and Spicy Cinnamon Rub

Directions:
Supply your smoker with wood pellets and follow the manufacturer's specific start-up procedure. Preheat the grill, with the lid closed, to 180°F.   Using your hands, work the rub into the turkey wings, coating them completely.   Place the wings directly on the grill grate and cook for 30 minutes.   Increase the grill's temperature to 325°F and continue to cook until the turkey's internal temperature reaches 170°F. Remove the wings from the grill and serve immediately.

235. Chicken Tenders

Servings: 2 To 4   Cooking Time: 1 Hour, 20 Minutes
Ingredients:
- 1 pound boneless, skinless chicken breast tenders
- 1 batch Chicken Rub

Directions:
Supply your smoker with wood pellets and follow the manufacturer's specific start-up procedure. Preheat the grill, with the lid closed, to 180°F.   Season the chicken tenders with the rub. Using your hands, work the rub into the meat.   Place the tenders directly on the grill grate and smoke for 1 hour.   Increase the grill's temperature to 300°F and continue to cook until the tenders' internal temperature reaches 170°F. Remove the tenders from the grill and serve immediately.

236. Traditional Bbq Chicken

Servings: 8   Cooking Time: 1 To 2 Hours
Ingredients:
- 8 boneless, skinless chicken breasts
- 2 teaspoons salt
- 2 teaspoons freshly ground black pepper
- 2 teaspoons garlic powder
- 2 cups The Ultimate BBQ Sauce or your preferred barbecue sauce, divided

Directions:
Supply your smoker with wood pellets and follow the manufacturer's specific start-up procedure. Preheat, with the lid closed, to 250°F.   Place the chicken breasts in a large pan and sprinkle both sides with the salt, pepper, and garlic powder, being sure to rub under the skin.   Place the roasting pan on the grill, close the lid, and smoke for 1 hour 30 minutes to 2 hours, or until a meat thermometer inserted in the thickest part of each breast reads 165°F. During the last 15 minutes of cooking, cover the chicken with 1 cup of barbecue sauce.   Serve the chicken warm with the remaining 1 cup of barbecue sauce.

237. Thanksgiving Dinner Turkey

Servings: 16   Cooking Time: 4 Hours
Ingredients:
- ½ lb. butter, softened
- 2 tbsp. fresh thyme, chopped
- 2 tbsp. fresh rosemary, chopped
- 6 garlic cloves, crushed
- 1 (20-lb.) whole turkey, neck and giblets removed
- Salt and freshly ground black pepper, to taste

Directions:
Set the temperature of   Grill to 300 degrees F and preheat with closed lid for 15 minutes, using charcoal. In a bowl, place butter, fresh herbs, garlic, salt and black pepper and mix well.   With your fingers, separate the turkey skin from breast to create a pocket.   Stuff the breast pocket with ¼-inch thick layer of butter mixture. Season the turkey with salt and black pepper evenly. Arrange the turkey onto the grill and cook for 3-4 hours.

Remove the turkey from grill and place onto a cutting board for about 15-20 minutes before carving. With a sharp knife, cut the turkey into desired-sized pieces and serve.

Nutrition Info: Calories per serving: 965; Carbohydrates: 0.6g; Protein: 106.5g; Fat: 52g; Sugar: 0g; Sodium: 1916mg; Fiber: 0.2g

238. Buffalo Chicken Flatbread

Servings: 6   Cooking Time: 30 Minutes
Ingredients:
- 6 mini pita bread
- 1-1/2 cups buffalo sauce
- 4 cups chicken breasts, cooked and cubed
- 3 cups mozzarella cheese
- Blue cheese for drizzling

Directions:
Preheat the wood pellet grill to 375-400°F. Place the breads on a flat surface and evenly spread sauce over all of them. Toss the chicken with the remaining buffalo sauce and place it on the pita breads. Top with cheese then place the breads on the grill but indirectly from the heat. Close the grill lid. Cook for 7 minutes or until the cheese has melted and the edges are toasty. Remove from grill and drizzle with blue cheese. Serve and enjoy.

Nutrition Info: Calories: 254 Cal Fat: 13 g Carbohydrates: 4 g   Protein: 33 g Fiber: 3 g

239. Turkey Legs

Servings: 4   Cooking Time: 5 Hours
Ingredients:
- 4 turkey legs
- For the Brine:
- 1/2 cup curing salt
- 1 tablespoon whole black peppercorns
- 1 cup BBQ rub
- 1/2 cup brown sugar
- 2 bay leaves
- 2 teaspoons liquid smoke
- 16 cups of warm water
- 4 cups ice
- 8 cups of cold water

Directions:
Prepare the brine and for this, take a large stockpot, place it over high heat, pour warm water in it, add peppercorn, bay leaves, and liquid smoke, stir in salt, sugar, and BBQ rub and bring it to a boil. Remove pot from heat, bring it to room temperature, then pour in cold water, add ice cubes and let the brine chill in the refrigerator. Then add turkey legs in it, submerge them completely, and let soak for 24 hours in the refrigerator. After 24 hours, remove turkey legs from the brine, rinse well and pat dry with paper towels. When ready to cook, switch on the grill, fill the grill hopper with hickory flavored wood pellets, power the grill on by using the control panel, select 'smoke' on the temperature dial, or set the temperature to 250 degrees F and let it preheat for a minimum of 15 minutes. When the grill has preheated,

open the lid, place turkey legs on the grill grate, shut the grill, and smoke for 5 hours until nicely browned and the internal temperature reaches 165 degrees F. Serve immediately.

Nutrition Info: Calories: 416 Cal ;Fat: 13.3 g ;Carbs: 0 g ;Protein: 69.8 g ;Fiber: 0 g

240. Smoked Quarters

Servings: 2 To 4   Cooking Time: 2 Hours
Ingredients:
- 4 chicken quarters
- 2 tablespoons olive oil
- 1 batch Chicken Rub
- 2 tablespoons butter

Directions:
Supply your smoker with wood pellets and follow the manufacturer's specific start-up procedure. Preheat the grill, with the lid closed, to 180°F. Coat the chicken quarters all over with olive oil and season them with the rub. Using your hands, work the rub into the meat. Place the quarters directly on the grill grate and smoke for 1½ hours. Baste the quarters with the butter and increase the grill's temperature to 375°F. Continue to cook until the chicken's internal temperature reaches 170°F. Remove the quarters from the grill and let them rest for 10 minutes before serving.

241. Smoked Airline Chicken

Servings: 4   Cooking Time: 1 To 2 Hours
Ingredients:
- 2 boneless chicken breasts with drumettes attached
- ½ cup soy sauce
- ½ cup teriyaki sauce
- ¼ cup canola oil
- ¼ cup white vinegar
- 1 tablespoon minced garlic
- ¼ cup chopped scallions
- 2 teaspoons freshly ground black pepper
- 1 teaspoon ground mustard

Directions:
Place the chicken in a baking dish. In a bowl, whisk together the soy sauce, teriyaki sauce, canola oil, vinegar, garlic, scallions, pepper and ground mustard, then pour this marinade over the chicken, coating both sides. Refrigerate the chicken in marinade for 4 hours, turning over every hour. When ready to smoke the chicken, supply your smoker with wood pellets and follow the manufacturer's specific start-up procedure. Preheat, with the lid closed, to 250°F. Remove the chicken from the marinade but do not rinse. Discard the marinade. Arrange the chicken directly on the grill, close the lid, and smoke for 1 hour 30 minutes to 2 hours, or until a meat thermometer inserted in the thickest part of the meat reads 165°F. Let the meat rest for 3 minutes before serving.

242. Teriyaki Wings

Servings: 8   Cooking Time: 50 Minutes
Ingredients:
- 2 ½ pounds large chicken wings
- 1 tablespoon toasted sesame seeds
- For the Marinade:
- 2 scallions, sliced
- 2 tablespoons grated ginger
- ½ teaspoon minced garlic
- 1/4 cup brown sugar
- 1/2 cup soy sauce
- 2 tablespoon rice wine vinegar
- 2 teaspoons sesame oil
- 1/4 cup water

Directions:
Prepare the chicken wings and for this, remove tips from the wings, cut each chicken wing through the joint into three pieces, and then place in a large plastic bag. Prepare the sauce and for this, take a small saucepan, place it over medium-high heat, add all of its ingredients in it, stir until mixed, and bring it to a boil.   Then switch heat to medium level, simmer the sauce for 10 minutes, and when done, cool the sauce completely. Pour the sauce over chicken wings, seal the bag, turn it upside down to coat chicken wings with the sauce and let it marinate for a minimum of 8 hours in the refrigerator. When ready to cook, switch on the grill, fill the grill hopper with maple-flavored wood pellets, power the grill on by using the control panel, select 'smoke' on the temperature dial, or set the temperature to 350 degrees F and let it preheat for a minimum of 15 minutes. Meanwhile,   When the grill has preheated, open the lid, place chicken wings on the grill grate, shut the grill and smoke for 50 minutes until crispy and meat is no longer pink, turning halfway.   When done, transfer chicken wings to a dish, sprinkle with sesame seeds and then serve.
Nutrition Info: Calories: 150 Cal ;Fat: 7.5 g ;Carbs: 6 g ;Protein: 12 g ;Fiber: 1 g

243. Roasted Chicken With Pimenton Potatoes

Servings: 16   Cooking Time: 1 Hour
Ingredients:
- 2 whole chicken
- 6 clove garlic, minced
- 2 tablespoons salt
- 3 tablespoons pimento (smoked paprika)
- 3 tablespoons extra virgin olive oil
- 2 bunch fresh thyme
- 3 pounds Yukon gold potatoes

Directions:
Season the whole chicken with garlic, salt, paprika, olive oil, and thyme. Massage the chicken to coat all surface of the chicken with the spices. Tie the legs together with a string. Place in a baking dish and place the potatoes on the side. Season the potatoes with salt and olive oil. Allow the chicken to rest in the fridge for 4 hours.

When ready to cook, fire the   Grill to 300F. Use preferred wood pellets. Close the grill lid and preheat for 15 minutes.   Place the chicken and potatoes in the grill and cook for 1 hour until a thermometer inserted in the thickest part of the chicken comes out clean. Remove from the grill and allow to rest before carving.
Nutrition Info: Calories per serving: 210; Protein: 26.1g; Carbs: 15.3g; Fat: 4.4g Sugar: 0.7g

244. Wild West Wings

Servings: 4   Cooking Time: 1 Hour
Ingredients:
- 2 pounds chicken wings
- 2 tablespoons extra-virgin olive oil
- 2 packages ranch dressing mix (such as Hidden Valley brand)
- ¼ cup prepared ranch dressing (optional)

Directions:
Supply your smoker with wood pellets and follow the manufacturer's specific start-up procedure. Preheat, with the lid closed, to 350°F.   Place the chicken wings in a large bowl and toss with the olive oil and ranch dressing mix.   Arrange the wings directly on the grill, or line the grill with aluminum foil for easy cleanup, close the lid, and smoke for 25 minutes.   Flip and smoke for 20 to 35 minutes more, or until a meat thermometer inserted in the thickest part of the wings reads 165°F and the wings are crispy. (Note: The wings will likely be done after 45 minutes, but an extra 10 to 15 minutes makes them crispy without drying the meat.)   Serve warm with ranch dressing (if using).

245. Lemon Chicken

Servings: 6   Cooking Time: 10 Minutes
Ingredients:
- 2 teaspoons honey
- 1 tablespoon lemon juice
- 1 teaspoon lemon zest
- 1 clove garlic, coarsely chopped
- 2 sprigs thyme
- Salt and pepper to taste
- ½ cup olive oil
- 6 chicken breast fillets

Directions:
Mix the honey, lemon juice, lemon zest, garlic, thyme, salt and pepper in a bowl.   Gradually add olive oil to the mixture.   Soak the chicken fillets in the mixture. Cover and refrigerate for 4 hours.   Preheat the wood pellet grill to 400 degrees F for 15 minutes while the lid is closed.   Grill the chicken for 5 minutes per side. Tips: You can also make additional marinade to be used for basting during grill time.

246. Jamaican Jerk Chicken Quarters

Servings: 4   Cooking Time: 1 To 2 Hours
Ingredients:

- 4 chicken leg quarters, scored
- ¼ cup canola oil
- ½ cup Jamaican Jerk Paste
- 1 tablespoon whole allspice (pimento) berries

Directions:
Supply your smoker with wood pellets and follow the manufacturer's specific start-up procedure. Preheat, with the lid closed, to 275°F. Brush the chicken with canola oil, then brush 6 tablespoons of the Jerk paste on and under the skin. Reserve the remaining 2 tablespoons of paste for basting. Throw the whole allspice berries in with the wood pellets for added smoke flavor. Arrange the chicken on the grill, close the lid, and smoke for 1 hour to 1 hour 30 minutes, or until a meat thermometer inserted in the thickest part of the thigh reads 165°F. Let the meat rest for 5 minutes and baste with the reserved jerk paste prior to serving.

247. Smoked Lemon Chicken Breasts

Servings: 6   Cooking Time: 30 Minutes
Ingredients:
- 2 lemons, zested and juiced
- 1 clove of garlic, minced
- 2 teaspoons honey
- 2 teaspoons salt
- 1 teaspoon ground black pepper
- 2 sprigs fresh thyme
- ½ cup olive oil
- 6 boneless chicken breasts

Directions:
Place all ingredients in a bowl. Massage the chicken breasts so that it is coated with the marinade. Place in the fridge to marinate for at least 4 hours. Fire the Grill to 350F. Use apple wood pellets. Close the grill lid and preheat for 15 minutes. Place the chicken breasts on the grill grate and cook for 15 minutes on both sides. Serve immediately or drizzle with lemon juice.

Nutrition Info: Calories per serving: 671 ; Protein: 60.6 g; Carbs: 3.5 g; Fat: 44.9g Sugar: 2.3g

248. Serrano Chicken Wings

Servings: 4   Cooking Time: 40 Minutes
Ingredients:
- 4 lb. chicken wings
- 2 cups beer
- 2 teaspoons crushed red pepper
- Cajun seasoning powder
- 1 lb. Serrano chili peppers
- 1 teaspoon fresh basil
- 1 teaspoon dried oregano
- 4 cloves garlic
- 1 cup vinegar
- Salt and pepper to taste

Directions:
Soak the chicken wings in beer. Sprinkle with crushed red pepper. Cover and refrigerate for 12 hours. Remove chicken from brine. Season with Cajun seasoning. Preheat your wood pellet grill to 325 degrees F for 15 minutes while the lid is closed. Add the chicken wings and Serrano chili peppers on the grill. Grill for 5 minutes per side. Remove chili peppers and place in a food processor. Grill the chicken for another 20 minutes. Add the rest of the ingredients to the food processor. Pulse until smooth. Dip the chicken wings in the sauce. Grill for 5 minutes and serve.
Tips: You can also use prepared pepper sauce to save time.

249. Hellfire Chicken Wings

Servings: 6   Cooking Time: 40 Minutes
Ingredients:
- 3 pounds chicken wings, tips removed
- 2 tablespoons olive oil
- For the Rub:
- 1 teaspoon onion powder
- 1 teaspoon salt
- 1 teaspoon garlic powder
- 1 tablespoon paprika
- 1 teaspoon ground black pepper
- 1 teaspoon celery seed
- 1 teaspoon cayenne pepper
- 2 teaspoons brown sugar
- For the Sauce:
- 4 jalapeno peppers, sliced crosswise
- 8 tablespoons butter, unsalted
- 1/2 cup hot sauce
- 1/2 cup cilantro leaves

Directions:
Switch on the grill, fill the grill hopper with hickory flavored wood pellets, power the grill on by using the control panel, select 'smoke' on the temperature dial, or set the temperature to 350 degrees F and let it preheat for a minimum of 15 minutes. Prepare the chicken wings and for this, remove tips from the wings, cut each chicken wing through the joint into two pieces, and then place in a large bowl. Prepare the rub and for this, take a small bowl, place all of its ingredients in it and then stir until combined. Sprinkle prepared rub on the chicken wings and then toss until well coated. Meanwhile, When the grill has preheated, open the lid, place chicken wings on the grill grate, shut the grill and smoke for 40 minutes until golden brown and skin have turned crisp, turning halfway. Meanwhile, prepare the sauce and for this, take a small saucepan, place it over medium-low heat, add butter in it and when it melts, add jalapeno and cook for 4 minutes. Then stir in hot sauce and cilantro until mixed and remove the pan from heat. When done, transfer chicken wings to a dish, top with prepared sauce, toss until coated, and then serve.

Nutrition Info: Calories: 250 Cal ;Fat: 15 g ;Carbs: 11 g ;Protein: 19 g ;Fiber: 1 g

250. Smoked Chicken Drumsticks

Servings: 5   Cooking Time: 2 Hours 30 Minutes
Ingredients:
- 10 chicken drumsticks

- 2tsp garlic powder
- 1tsp salt
- 1tsp onion powder
- 1/2 tsp ground black pepper
- ½ tsp cayenne pepper
- 1tsp brown sugar
- 1/3 cup hot sauce
- 1tsp paprika
- ½ tsp thyme

Directions:
In a large mixing bowl, combine the garlic powder, sugar, hot sauce, paprika, thyme, cayenne, salt, and ground pepper. Add the drumsticks and toss to combine. Cover the bowl and refrigerate for 1 hour.   Remove the drumsticks from the marinade and let them sit for about 1 hour until they are at room temperature.   Arrange the drumsticks into a rack.   Start your pellet grill on smoke, leaving the lid open for 5 minutes for the fire to start.   Close the lid and preheat grill to 250°F, using hickory or apple hardwood pellets.   Place the rack on the grill and smoke drumsticks for 2 hours, 30 minutes, or until the drumsticks' internal temperature reaches 180°F.   Remove drumsticks from heat and let them rest for a few minutes.   Serve.
Nutrition Info: Calories: 167 Total Fat: 5.4 g Saturated Fat: 1.4 g Cholesterol: 81 mg Sodium: 946 mg Total Carbohydrate: 2.6 g Dietary Fiber: 0.5 g Total Sugars: 1.3 g Protein: 25.7 g

251. Chicken Tikka Masala

Servings: 4   Cooking Time: 1 Hour
Ingredients:
- 1 tablespoon garam masala
- 1 tablespoon smoked paprika
- 1 tablespoon ground coriander
- 1 tablespoon ground cumin
- 1 teaspoon ground cayenne pepper
- 1 teaspoon turmeric
- 1 onion, sliced
- 6 cloves garlic, minced
- 1/4 cup olive oil
- 1 tablespoon ginger, chopped
- 1 tablespoon lemon juice
- 1 1/2 cups Greek yogurt
- 1 tablespoon lime juice
- 1 tablespoon curry powder
- Salt to taste
- 1 tablespoon lime juice
- 12 chicken drumsticks
- Chopped cilantro

Directions:
Make the marinade by mixing all the spices, onion, garlic, olive oil, ginger, lemon juice, yogurt, lime juice, curry powder and salt.   Transfer to a food processor. Pulse until smooth.   Divide the mixture into two. Marinade the chicken in the first bowl.   Cover the bowl and refrigerate for 12 hours.   Set the   wood pellet grill to high.   Preheat it for 15 minutes while the lid is closed. Grill the chicken for 50 minutes.   Garnish with the

chopped cilantro.   Tips: You can also smoke the chicken before grilling.

252. Spatchcocked Turkey

Servings: 10 To 14   Cooking Time: 2 Hours
Ingredients:
- 1 whole turkey
- 2 tablespoons olive oil
- 1 batch Chicken Rub

Directions:
Supply your smoker with wood pellets and follow the manufacturer's specific start-up procedure. Preheat the grill, with the lid closed, to 350°F.   To remove the turkey's backbone, place the turkey on a work surface, on its breast. Using kitchen shears, cut along one side of the turkey's backbone and then the other. Pull out the bone. Once the backbone is removed, turn the turkey breast-side up and flatten it.   Coat the turkey with olive oil and season it on both sides with the rub. Using your hands, work the rub into the meat and skin.   Place the turkey directly on the grill grate, breast-side up, and cook until its internal temperature reaches 170°F.   Remove the turkey from the grill and let it rest for 10 minutes, before carving and serving.

253. Trager Smoked Spatchcock Turkey

Servings: 8   Cooking Time: 1 Hour 15 Minutes;
Ingredients:
- 1 turkey
- 1/2 cup melted butter
- 1/4 cup   chicken rub
- 1 tbsp onion powder
- 1 tbsp garlic powder
- 1 tbsp rubbed sage

Directions:
Preheat your   to high temperature.   Place the turkey on a chopping board with the breast side down and the legs pointing towards you.   Cut either side of the turkey backbone, to remove the spine. Flip the turkey and place it on a pan   Season both sides with the seasonings and place it on the grill skin side up on the grill.   Cook for 30 minutes, reduce temperature, and cook for 45 more minutes or until the internal temperature reaches 165F.   Remove from the   and let rest for 15 minutes before slicing and serving.
Nutrition Info: Calories 156, Total fat 16g, Saturated fat 2g, Total carbs 1g, Net carbs 1g Protein 2g, Sugars 0g, Fiber 0g, Sodium 19mg

254. Paprika Chicken

Servings: 7   Cooking Time: 2 – 4 Hours
Ingredients:
- 4-6 chicken breast
- 4 tablespoons olive oil
- 2tablespoons smoked paprika
- ½ tablespoon salt

64

- ¼ teaspoon pepper
- 2 teaspoons garlic powder
- 2 teaspoons garlic salt
- 2 teaspoons pepper
- 1 teaspoon cayenne pepper
- 1 teaspoon rosemary

Directions:
Preheat your smoker to 220 degrees Fahrenheit using your favorite wood Pellets   Prepare your chicken breast according to your desired shapes and transfer to a greased baking dish   Take a medium bowl and add spices, stir well   Press the spice mix over chicken and transfer the chicken to smoker   Smoke for 1-1 and a ½ hours   Turn-over and cook for 30 minutes more Once the internal temperature reaches 165 degrees Fahrenheit   Remove from the smoker and cover with foil   Allow it to rest for 15 minutes   Enjoy!

Nutrition Info: Calories: 237 Fats: 6.1g Carbs: 14g Fiber: 3g

255. Cajun Chicken Breasts

Servings: 6   Cooking Time: 6 Hours
Ingredients:
- 2 lb. skinless, boneless chicken breasts
- 2 tbsp. Cajun seasoning
- 1 C. BBQ sauce

Directions:
Set the temperature of   Grill to 225 degrees F and preheat with closed lid for 15 minutes.   Rub the chicken breasts with Cajun seasoning generously. Place the chicken breasts onto the grill and cook for about 4-6 hours.   During last hour of cooking, coat the breasts with BBQ sauce twice.   Serve hot.

Nutrition Info: Calories per serving: 252; Carbohydrates: 15.1g; Protein: 33.8g; Fat: 5.5g; Sugar: 10.9g; Sodium: 570mg; Fiber: 0.3g

256. Beer Can Chicken

Servings: 6   Cooking Time: 1 Hour And 15 Minutes
Ingredients:
- 5-pound chicken
- 1/2 cup dry chicken rub
- 1 can beer

Directions:
Preheat your wood pellet grill on smoke for 5 minutes with the lid open.   The lid must then be closed and then preheated up to 450 degrees Fahrenheit   Pour out half of the beer then shove the can in the chicken and use the legs like a tripod.   Place the chicken on the grill until the internal temperature reaches 165°F.   Remove from the grill and let rest for 20 minutes before serving. Enjoy.

Nutrition Info: Calories: 882 Cal Fat: 51 g Carbohydrates: 2 g   Protein: 94 g Fiber: 0 g

257. Bourbon Bbq Smoked Chicken Wings

Servings: 8   Cooking Time: 24 Minutes
Ingredients:
- 4 pounds chicken wings, patted dry
- 2 tablespoons olive oil
- Salt and pepper to taste
- ½ medium yellow onions, minced
- 5 cloves garlic, mince
- ½ cup bourbon
- 2 cups ketchup
- 1/3 cup apple cider vinegar
- 2 tablespoons liquid smoke
- ½ teaspoon kosher salt
- ½ teaspoon black pepper
- A dash of hot sauce

Directions:
Place the chicken in a bowl and drizzle with olive oil. Season with salt and pepper to taste. In another bowl, combine the rest of the ingredients and set aside.   Fire the   Grill to 400F. Use hickory wood pellets. Close the lid and allow to preheat for 15 minutes.   Place the chicken on the grill grate and cook for 12 minutes on each side.   Using a brush, brush the chicken wings with bourbon sauce on all sides.   Flip the chicken and cook for another 12 minutes with the lid closed.

Nutrition Info: Calories per serving: 384 ; Protein: 50.7g; Carbs: 17.8 g; Fat: 11.5g Sugar: 13.1g

258. Smoked Turkey Breast

Servings: 2 To 4   Cooking Time: 1 To 2 Hours
Ingredients:
- 1 (3-pound) turkey breast
- Salt
- Freshly ground black pepper
- 1 teaspoon garlic powder

Directions:
Supply your smoker with wood pellets and follow the manufacturer's specific start-up procedure. Preheat the grill, with the lid closed, to 180°F.   Season the turkey breast all over with salt, pepper, and garlic powder. Place the breast directly on the grill grate and smoke for 1 hour.   Increase the grill's temperature to 350°F and continue to cook until the turkey's internal temperature reaches 170°F. Remove the breast from the grill and serve immediately.

259. Wood Pellet Grilled Chicken Kabobs

Servings: 6   Cooking Time: 12 Minutes
Ingredients:
- 1/2 cup olive oil
- 2 tbsp white vinegar
- 1 tbsp lemon juice
- 1-1/2 tbsp salt
- 1/2 tbsp pepper, coarsely ground
- 2 tbsp chives, freshly chopped
- 1-1/2 tbsp thyme, freshly chopped
- 2 tbsp Italian parsley freshly chopped

- 1tbsp garlic, minced
- Kabobs
- 1 each orange, red, and yellow pepper
- 1-1/2 pounds chicken breast, boneless and skinless
- 12 mini mushrooms

Directions:
In a mixing bowl, add all the marinade ingredients and mix well. Toss the chicken and mushrooms in the marinade then refrigerate for 30 minutes.   Meanwhile, soak the skewers in hot water. Remove the chicken from the fridge and start assembling the kabobs.   Preheat your wood pellet to 450°F.   Grill the kabobs in the wood pellet for 6 minutes, flip them and grill for 6 more minutes.   Remove from the grill and let rest. Heat up the naan bread on the grill for 2 minutes.   Serve and enjoy.

Nutrition Info: Calories: 165 Cal Fat: 13 g Carbohydrates: 1 g   Protein: 33 g Fiber: 0 g

260. Wood Pellet Chicken Breasts

Servings: 6   Cooking Time: 15 Minutes
Ingredients:
- 3 chicken breasts
- 1 tbsp avocado oil
- 1/4 tbsp garlic powder
- 1/4 tbsp onion powder
- 3/4 tbsp salt
- 1/4 tbsp pepper

Directions:
Preheat your pellet to 375°F.   Half the chicken breasts lengthwise then coat with avocado oil.   With the spices, drizzle it on all sides to season   Drizzle spices to season the chicken. Put the chicken on top of the grill and begin to cook until its internal temperature approaches 165 degrees Fahrenheit. Put the chicken on top of the grill and begin to cook until it rises to a temperature of 165 degrees Fahrenheit   Serve and enjoy.

Nutrition Info: Calories: 120 Cal Fat: 4 g Carbohydrates: 0 g   Protein: 19 g Fiber: 0 g

261. Korean Chicken Wings

Servings: 6   Cooking Time: 1 Hour
Ingredients:
- 3 pounds of chicken wings
- 2 tablespoons olive oil
- For the Brine:
- 1 head garlic, halved
- 1 lemon, halved
- 1/2 cup sugar
- 1 cup of sea salt
- 4 sprigs of thyme
- 10 peppercorns
- 16 cups of water
- For the Sauce:
- 2 teaspoons minced garlic
- 1/2 cup gochujang hot pepper paste
- 1 tablespoon grated ginger

- 2 tablespoons of rice wine vinegar
- 1/3 cup honey
- 1/4 cup soy sauce
- 2 tablespoons lime juice
- 2 tablespoons toasted sesame oil
- 1/4 cup melted butter

Directions:
Prepare the brine and for this, take a large stockpot, place it over high heat, pour in water, stir in salt and sugar until dissolved, and bring to a boil.   Then remove the pot from heat, add remaining ingredients for the brine, and bring the brine to room temperature.   Add chicken wings, submerge them completely, cover the pot and let wings soak for a minimum of 4 hours in the refrigerator. When ready to cook, switch on the   grill, fill the grill hopper with flavored wood pellets, power the grill on by using the control panel, select 'smoke' on the temperature dial, or set the temperature to 375 degrees F and let it preheat for a minimum of 15 minutes. Meanwhile, remove chicken wings from the brine, pat dry with paper towels, place them in a large bowl, drizzle with oil and toss until well coated.   When the grill has preheated, open the lid, place chicken wings on the grill grate, shut the grill, and smoke for 1 hour until the internal temperature reaches 165 degrees F. Meanwhile, prepare the sauce and for this, take a medium bowl, place all of the sauce ingredients in it and whisk until smooth.   When done, transfer chicken wings to a dish, top with prepared sauce, toss until coated, and then serve.

Nutrition Info: Calories: 137 Cal ;Fat: 9 g ;Carbs: 4 g ;Protein: 8 g ;Fiber: 1 g

262. Lemon Rosemary And Beer Marinated Chicken

Servings: 6   Cooking Time: 55 Minutes
Ingredients:
- 1 whole chicken
- 1 lemon, zested and juiced
- 1 teaspoon salt
- 1 teaspoon ground black pepper
- 1 teaspoon rosemary, chopped
- 12-ounce beer, apple-flavored

Directions:
Place all ingredients in a bowl and allow the chicken to marinate for at least 12 hours in the fridge.   When ready to cook, fire the   Grill to 350F. Use preferred wood pellets.   Close the grill lid and preheat for 15 minutes.   Place the chicken on the grill grate and cook for 55 minutes.   Cook until the internal temperature reads at 165F.   Take the chicken out and allow to rest before carving.

Nutrition Info: Calories per serving: 288; Protein: 36.1g; Carbs: 4.4g; Fat: 13.1g Sugar: 0.7g

263. Bacon-wrapped Chicken Tenders

Servings: 6   Cooking Time: 30 Minutes
Ingredients:

- 1-pound chicken tenders
- 10 strips bacon
- 1/2 tbsp Italian seasoning
- 1/2 tbsp black pepper
- 1/2 tbsp salt
- 1 tbsp paprika
- 1 tbsp onion powder
- 1 tbsp garlic powder
- 1/3 cup light brown sugar
- 1 tbsp chili powder

Directions:
Preheat your wood pellet smoker to 350°F. Mix seasonings Sprinkle the mixture on all sides of chicken tenders Wrap each chicken tender with a strip of bacon Mix sugar and chili then sprinkle the mixture on the bacon-wrapped chicken. Place them on the smoker and smoker for 30 minutes with the lid closed or until the chicken is cooked. Serve and enjoy.
Nutrition Info: Calories: 206 Cal Fat: 7.9 g Carbohydrates: 1.5 g Protein: 30.3 g Fiber: 0 g

264. Buttered Thanksgiving Turkey

Servings: 12 To 14   Cooking Time: 5 To 6 Hours
Ingredients:
- 1 whole turkey (make sure the turkey is not pre-brined)
- 2 batches Garlic Butter Injectable
- 3 tablespoons olive oil
- 1 batch Chicken Rub
- 2 tablespoons butter

Directions:
Supply your smoker with wood pellets and follow the manufacturer's specific start-up procedure. Preheat the grill, with the lid closed, to 180°F. Inject the turkey throughout with the garlic butter injectable. Coat the turkey with olive oil and season it with the rub. Using your hands, work the rub into the meat and skin. Place the turkey directly on the grill grate and smoke for 3 or 4 hours (for an 8- to 12-pound turkey, cook for 3 hours; for a turkey over 12 pounds, cook for 4 hours), basting it with butter every hour. Increase the grill's temperature to 375°F and continue to cook until the turkey's internal temperature reaches 170°F. Remove the turkey from the grill and let it rest for 10 minutes, before carving and serving.

265. Wood Pellet Grilled Buffalo Chicken

Servings: 6   Cooking Time: 20 Minutes
Ingredients:
- 5 chicken breasts, boneless and skinless
- 2 tbsp homemade bbq rub
- 1 cup homemade Cholula buffalo sauce

Directions:
Preheat the wood pellet grill to 400°F. Slice the chicken into long strips and season with bbq rub. Place the chicken on the grill and paint both sides with buffalo sauce. Cook for 4 minutes with the grill closed. Cook while flipping and painting with buffalo

sauce every 5 minutes until the internal temperature reaches 165°F. Remove from the grill and serve when warm. Enjoy.
Nutrition Info: Calories 176, Total fat 4g, Saturated fat 1g, Total carbs 1g, Net carbs 1g, Protein 32g, Sugar 1g, Fiber 0g, Sodium: 631mg

266. Chinese Inspired Duck Legs

Servings: 8   Cooking Time: 1 Hour 10 Minutes
Ingredients:
- For Glaze:
- ¼ C. fresh orange juice
- ¼ C. orange marmalade
- ¼ C. mirin
- 2 tbsp. hoisin sauce
- ½ tsp. red pepper flakes, crushed
- For Duck:
- 1 tsp. kosher salt
- ¾ tsp. freshly ground black pepper
- ¾ tsp. Chinese five-spice powder
- 8 (6-oz.) duck legs

Directions:
Set the temperature of Grill to 235 degrees F and preheat with closed lid for 15 minutes. Forb glaze: in a small pan, add all ingredients over medium-high heat and bring to gentle boil, stirring continuously. Remove from heat and set aside. For rub: in a small bowl, mix together salt, black pepper and five-spice powder. Rub the duck legs with spice rub evenly. Place the duck legs onto the grill, skin side up and cook for about 50 minutes. Coat the duck legs with glaze ad cook for about 20 minutes, flipping and coating with glaze after every 5 minutes.
Nutrition Info: Calories per serving: 303; Carbohydrates: 0.1g; Protein: 49.5g; Fat: 10.2g; Sugar: 0g; Sodium: 474mg; Fiber: 0.1g

267. Sweet Sriracha Bbq Chicken

Servings: 5   Cooking Time: 1 And ½-2 Hours
Ingredients:
- 1cup sriracha
- ½ cup butter
- ½ cup molasses
- ½ cup ketchup
- ¼ cup firmly packed brown sugar
- 1teaspoon salt
- 1teaspoon fresh ground black pepper
- 1whole chicken, cut into pieces
- ½ teaspoon fresh parsley leaves, chopped

Directions:
Preheat your smoker to 250 degrees Fahrenheit using cherry wood Take a medium saucepan and place it over low heat, stir in butter, sriracha, ketchup, molasses, brown sugar, mustard, pepper and salt and keep stirring until the sugar and salt dissolves Divide the sauce into two portions Brush the chicken half with the sauce and reserve the remaining for serving Make sure to keep the sauce for serving on the side, and keep the other

portion for basting   Transfer chicken to your smoker rack and smoke for about 1 and a ½ to 2 hours until the internal temperature reaches 165 degrees Fahrenheit   Sprinkle chicken with parsley and serve with reserved BBQ sauce   Enjoy!

Nutrition Info: Calories: 148 Fats: 0.6g Carbs: 10g Fiber: 1g

268. Smoked Chicken Thighs

Servings: 6   Cooking Time: 24 Minutes.
Ingredients:
- 6 chicken thighs
- ½ cup commercial BBQ sauce of your choice
- 1 ½ tablespoon poultry spice
- 4 tablespoons butter

Directions:
Place all ingredients in a bowl except for the butter. Massage the chicken to make sure that the chicken is coated with the marinade.   Place in the fridge to marinate for 4 hours.   Fire the   Grill to 350F. Use hickory wood pellets. Close the lid and preheat for 15 minutes.   When ready to cook, place the chicken on the grill grate and cook for 12 minutes on each side. Before serving the chicken, brush with butter on top.

Nutrition Info: Calories per serving: 504; Protein: 32.4g; Carbs: 2.7g; Fat: 39.9g Sugar: 0.9g

269. Smoking Duck With Mandarin Glaze

Servings: 4   Cooking Time: 4 Hours
Ingredients:
- 1 quart buttermilk
- 1 (5-pound) whole duck
- ¾ cup soy sauce
- ½ cup hoisin sauce
- ½ cup rice wine vinegar
- 2 tablespoons sesame oil
- 1 tablespoon freshly ground black pepper
- 1 tablespoon minced garlic
- Mandarin Glaze, for drizzling

Directions:
With a very sharp knife, remove as much fat from the duck as you can. Refrigerate or freeze the fat for later use. Pour the buttermilk into a large container with a lid and submerge the whole duck in it. Cover and let brine in the refrigerator for 4 to 6 hours.   Supply your smoker with wood pellets and follow the manufacturer's specific start-up procedure. Preheat, with the lid closed, to 250°F. Remove the duck from the buttermilk brine, then rinse it and pat dry with paper towels.   In a bowl, combine the soy sauce, hoisin sauce, vinegar, sesame oil, pepper, and garlic to form a paste. Reserve ¼ cup for basting. Poke holes in the skin of the duck and rub the remaining paste all over and inside the cavity.   Place the duck on the grill breast-side down, close the lid, and smoke for about 4 hours, basting every hour with the reserved paste, until a meat thermometer inserted in the thickest part of the meat reads 165°F. Use aluminum foil to tent the duck

in the last 30 minutes or so if it starts to brown too quickly.   To finish, drizzle with glaze.

270. Garlic Parmesan Chicken Wings

Servings: 6   Cooking Time: 20 Minutes
Ingredients:
- 5 pounds of chicken wings
- 1/2 cup chicken rub
- 3 tablespoons chopped parsley
- 1 cup shredded parmesan cheese
- For the Sauce:
- 5 teaspoons minced garlic
- 2 tablespoons chicken rub
- 1 cup butter, unsalted

Directions:
Switch on the   grill, fill the grill hopper with cherry flavored wood pellets, power the grill on by using the control panel, select 'smoke' on the temperature dial, or set the temperature to 450 degrees F and let it preheat for a minimum of 15 minutes.   Meanwhile, take a large bowl, place chicken wings in it, sprinkle with chicken rub and toss until well coated.   When the grill has preheated, open the lid, place chicken wings on the grill grate, shut the grill, and smoke for 10 minutes per side until the internal temperature reaches 165 degrees F. Meanwhile, prepare the sauce and for this, take a medium saucepan, place it over medium heat, add all the ingredients for the sauce in it and cook for 10 minutes until smooth, set aside until required.   When done, transfer chicken wings to a dish, top with prepared sauce, toss until mixed, garnish with cheese and parsley and then serve.

Nutrition Info: Calories: 180 Cal ;Fat: 1 g ;Carbs: 8 g ;Protein: 0 g ;Fiber: 0 g

271. Easy Smoked Chicken Breasts

Servings: 4   Cooking Time: 30 Minutes
Ingredients:
- 4 large chicken breasts, bones and skin removed
- 1 tablespoon olive oil
- 2 tablespoons brown sugar
- 2 tablespoons maple syrup
- 1 teaspoon celery seeds
- 2 tablespoons paprika
- 2 tablespoons salt
- 1 teaspoon black pepper
- 2 tablespoons garlic powder
- 2 tablespoons onion powder

Directions:
Place all ingredients in a bowl and massage the chicken with your hands. Place in the fridge to marinate for at least 4 hours.   Fire the   Grill to 350F and use maple wood pellets. Close the lid and allow to preheat to 15 minutes.   Place the chicken on the grill a and cook for 15 minutes with the lid closed.   Turn the chicken over and cook for another 10 minutes.   Insert a thermometer into the thickest part of the chicken and make sure that the temperature reads to 165F.

Remove the chicken from the grill and allow to rest for 5 minutes before slicing.

Nutrition Info: Calories per serving: 327 ; Protein: 40 g; Carbs: 23g; Fat: 9g Sugar: 13g

272. Smo-fried Chicken

Servings: 4 To 6   Cooking Time: 55 Minutes
Ingredients:
- 1 egg, beaten
- ½ cup milk
- 1 cup all-purpose flour
- 2 tablespoons salt
- 1 tablespoon freshly ground black pepper
- 2 teaspoons freshly ground white pepper
- 2 teaspoons cayenne pepper
- 2 teaspoons garlic powder
- 2 teaspoons onion powder
- 1 teaspoon smoked paprika
- 8 tablespoons (1 stick) unsalted butter, melted
- 1 whole chicken, cut up into pieces

Directions:
Supply your smoker with wood pellets and follow the manufacturer's specific start-up procedure. Preheat, with the lid closed, to 375°F.   In a medium bowl, combine the beaten egg with the milk and set aside.   In a separate medium bowl, stir together the flour, salt, black pepper, white pepper, cayenne, garlic powder, onion powder, and smoked paprika.   Line the bottom and sides of a high-sided metal baking pan with aluminum foil to ease cleanup.   Pour the melted butter into the prepared pan.   Dip the chicken pieces one at a time in the egg mixture, and then coat well with the seasoned flour. Transfer to the baking pan.   Smoke the chicken in the pan of butter ("smo-fry") on the grill, with the lid closed, for 25 minutes, then reduce the heat to 325°F and turn the chicken pieces over.   Continue smoking with the lid closed for about 30 minutes, or until a meat thermometer inserted in the thickest part of each chicken piece reads 165°F.   Serve immediately.

273. Wood Pellet Sheet Pan Chicken Fajitas

Servings: 10   Cooking Time: 10 Minutes
Ingredients:
- 2 tbsp oil
- 2 tbsp chile margarita seasoning
- 1 tbsp salt
- 1/2 tbsp onion powder
- 1/2 tbsp garlic, granulated
- 2-pound chicken breast, thinly sliced
- 1 red bell pepper, seeded and sliced
- 1 orange bell pepper
- 1 onion, sliced

Directions:
Preheat the wood pellet to 450°F. Meanwhile, mix oil and seasoning then toss the chicken and the peppers. Line a sheet pan with foil then place it in the preheated grill. Let it heat for 10 minutes with the grill's lid closed. Open the grill and place the chicken with the veggies on

the pan in a single layer. Cook for 10 minutes or until the chicken is cooked and no longer pink. Remove from grill and serve with tortilla or your favorite fixings.

Nutrition Info: Calories: 211 Cal Fat: 6 g Carbohydrates: 5 g   Protein: 29 g Fiber: 1 g

274. Wood Pellet Grilled Chicken

Servings: 6   Cooking Time: 1 Hour And 10 Minutes
Ingredients:
- 5 pounds whole chicken
- 1/2 cup oil
- Chicken rub

Directions:
Preheat your wood pellet on smoke with the lid open for 5 minutes. Close the lid, increase the temperature to 450°F and preheat for 15 more minutes.   Tie the chicken legs together with the baker's twine then rub the chicken with oil and coat with chicken rub.   Place the chicken on the grill with the breast side up.   Grill the chicken for 70 minutes without opening it or until the internal temperature reaches 165°F.   Once the chicken is out of the grill let it cool down for 15 minutes   Enjoy.

Nutrition Info: Calories: 935 Cal Fat: 53 g Carbohydrates: 0 g   Protein: 107 g Fiber: 0 g

275. Wood Pellet Smoked Spatchcock Turkey

Servings: 6   Cooking Time: 1 Hour 45 Minutes
Ingredients:
- 1 whole turkey
- 1/2 cup oil
- 1/4 cup chicken rub
- 1 tbsp onion powder
- 1 tbsp garlic powder
- 1 tbsp rubbed sage

Directions:
Preheat your wood pellet grill to high.   Meanwhile, place the turkey on a platter with the breast side down then cut on either side of the backbone to remove the spine.   Flip the turkey and season on both sides then place it on the preheated grill or on a pan if you want to catch the drippings.   Grill on high for 30 minutes, reduce the temperature to 325°F, and grill for 45 more minutes or until the internal temperature reaches 165°F Remove from the grill and let rest for 20 minutes before slicing and serving. Enjoy.

Nutrition Info: Calories 156, Total fat 16g, Saturated fat 2g, Total Carbs 1g, Net Carbs 1g, Protein 2g, Sugar 0g, Fiber 0g, Sodium: 19mg

276. Wood Pellet Grilled Buffalo Chicken

Servings: 6   Cooking Time: 20 Minutes
Ingredients:
- 5 chicken breasts, boneless and skinless
- 2 tbsp homemade barbeque rub
- 1 cup homemade Cholula buffalo sauce

Directions:
Preheat the wood pellet grill to 400°F. Slice the chicken into long strips and season with barbeque rub. Place the chicken on the grill and paint both sides with buffalo sauce. Cook for 4 minutes with the grill closed. Cook while flipping and painting with buffalo sauce every 5 minutes until the internal temperature reaches 165°F. Remove from the grill and serve when warm. Enjoy.
Nutrition Info: Calories: 176 Cal Fat: 4 g Carbohydrates: 1 g   Protein: 32 g Fiber: 0 g

277. Mini Turducken Roulade

Servings: 6   Cooking Time: 2 Hours
Ingredients:
- 1 (16-ounce) boneless turkey breast
- 1 (8-to 10-ounce) boneless duck breast
- 1 (8-ounce) boneless, skinless chicken breast
- Salt
- Freshly ground black pepper
- 2 cups Italian dressing
- 2 tablespoons Cajun seasoning
- 1 cup prepared seasoned stuffing mix
- 8 slices bacon
- Butcher's string

Directions:
Butterfly the turkey, duck, and chicken breasts, cover with plastic wrap and, using a mallet, flatten each ½ inch thick. Season all the meat on both sides with a little salt and pepper. In a medium bowl, combine the Italian dressing and Cajun seasoning. Spread one-fourth of the mixture on top of the flattened turkey breast. Place the duck breast on top of the turkey, spread it with one-fourth of the dressing mixture, and top with the stuffing mix. Place the chicken breast on top of the duck and spread with one-fourth of the dressing mixture. Supply your smoker with wood pellets and follow the manufacturer's specific start-up procedure. Preheat, with the lid closed, to 275°F. Tightly roll up the stack, tie with butcher's string, and slather the whole thing with the remaining dressing mixture. Wrap the bacon slices around the turducken and secure with toothpicks, or try making a bacon weave (see the technique for this in the Jalapeño-Bacon Pork Tenderloin recipe). Place the turducken roulade in a roasting pan. Transfer to the grill, close the lid, and roast for 2 hours, or until a meat thermometer inserted in the turducken reads 165°F. Tent with aluminum foil in the last 30 minutes, if necessary, to keep from overbrowning. Let the turducken rest for 15 to 20 minutes before carving. Serve warm.

278. Maple And Bacon Chicken

Servings: 7   Cooking Time: 1 And ½ Hours
Ingredients:
- 4 boneless and skinless chicken breast
- Salt as needed
- Fresh pepper

- 12 slices bacon, uncooked
- 1cup maple syrup
- ½ cup melted butter
- 1teaspoon liquid smoke

Directions:
Preheat your smoker to 250 degrees Fahrenheit Season the chicken with pepper and salt Wrap the breast with 3 bacon slices and cover the entire surface Secure the bacon with toothpicks Take a medium-sized bowl and stir in maple syrup, butter, liquid smoke, and mix well Reserve 1/3rd of this mixture for later use Submerge the chicken breast into the butter mix and coat them well Place a pan in your smoker and transfer the chicken to your smoker Smoker for 1 to 1 and a ½ hours Brush the chicken with reserved butter and smoke for 30 minutes more until the internal temperature reaches 165 degrees Fahrenheit Enjoy!
Nutrition Info: Calories: 458 Fats: 20g Carbs: 65g Fiber: 1g

279. Ultimate Tasty Chicken

Servings: 5   Cooking Time: 3 Hours
Ingredients:
- For Brine:
- 1 C. brown sugar
- ½ C. kosher salt
- 16 C. water
- For Chicken:
- 1 (3-lb.) whole chicken
- 1 tbsp. garlic, crushed
- 1 tsp. onion powder
- Salt and freshly ground black pepper, to taste
- 1 medium yellow onion, quartered
- 3 whole garlic cloves, peeled
- 1 lemon, quartered
- 4-5 fresh thyme sprigs

Directions:
For brine: in a bucket, dissolve brown sugar and kosher salt in water. Place the chicken in brine and refrigerate overnight. Set the temperature of Grill to 225 degrees F and preheat with closed lid for 15 minutes. Remove the chicken from brine and with paper towels, pat it dry. In a small bowl, mix together crushed garlic, onion powder, salt and black pepper. Rub the chicken with garlic mixture evenly. Stuff the cavity of chicken with onion, garlic cloves, lemon and thyme. With kitchen strings, tie the legs together. Place the chicken onto grill and cook, covered for about 2½-3 hours. Remove chicken from pallet grill and transfer onto a cutting board for about 10 minutes before carving. With a sharp knife, cut the chicken in desired sized pieces and serve.
Nutrition Info: Calories per serving: 641; Carbohydrates: 31.7g; Protein: 79.2g; Fat: 20.2g; Sugar: 29.3g; Sodium: 11500mg; Fiber: 0.6g

280. Applewood-smoked Whole Turkey

Servings: 6 To 8   Cooking Time: 5 To 6 Hours
Ingredients:
- 1 (10- to 12-pound) turkey, giblets removed
- Extra-virgin olive oil, for rubbing
- ¼ cup poultry seasoning
- 8 tablespoons (1 stick) unsalted butter, melted
- ½ cup apple juice
- 2 teaspoons dried sage
- 2 teaspoons dried thyme

Directions:
Supply your smoker with wood pellets and follow the manufacturer's specific start-up procedure. Preheat, with the lid closed, to 250°F.   Rub the turkey with oil and season with the poultry seasoning inside and out, getting under the skin.   In a bowl, combine the melted butter, apple juice, sage, and thyme to use for basting. Put the turkey in a roasting pan, place on the grill, close the lid, and grill for 5 to 6 hours, basting every hour, until the skin is brown and crispy, or until a meat thermometer inserted in the thickest part of the thigh reads 165°F.   Let the bird rest for 15 to 20 minutes before carving.

281. Smoke-roasted Chicken Thighs

Servings: 12 To 15   Cooking Time: 1 To 2 Hours
Ingredients:
- 3 pounds chicken thighs
- 2 teaspoons salt
- 2 teaspoons freshly ground black pepper
- 2 teaspoons garlic powder
- 2 teaspoons onion powder
- 2 cups prepared Italian dressing

Directions:
Place the chicken thighs in a shallow dish and sprinkle with the salt, pepper, garlic powder, and onion powder, being sure to get under the skin.   Cover with the Italian dressing, coating all sides, and refrigerate for 1 hour. Supply your smoker with wood pellets and follow the manufacturer's specific start-up procedure. Preheat, with the lid closed, to 250°F.   Remove the chicken thighs from the marinade and place directly on the grill, skin-side down. Discard the marinade.   Close the lid and roast the chicken for 1 hour 30 minutes to 2 hours, or until a meat thermometer inserted in the thickest part of the thighs reads 165°F. Do not turn the thighs during the smoking process.

282. Bbq Sauce Smothered Chicken Breasts

Servings: 4   Cooking Time: 30 Minutes
Ingredients:
- 1 tsp. garlic, crushed
- ¼ C. olive oil
- 1 tbsp. Worcestershire sauce
- 1 tbsp. sweet mesquite seasoning
- 4 chicken breasts
- 2 tbsp. regular BBQ sauce
- 2 tbsp. spicy BBQ sauce
- 2 tbsp. honey bourbon BBQ sauce

Directions:
Set the temperature of   Grill to 450 degrees F and preheat with closed lid for 15 minutes.   In a large bowl, mix together garlic, oil, Worcestershire sauce and mesquite seasoning.   Coat chicken breasts with seasoning mixture evenly.   Place the chicken breasts onto the grill and cook for about 20-30 minutes. Meanwhile, in a bowl, mix together all 3 BBQ sauces. In the last 4-5 minutes of cooking, coat breast with BBQ sauce mixture.   Serve hot.

Nutrition Info: Calories per serving: 421; Carbohydrates: 10.1g; Protein: 41,2g; Fat: 23.3g; Sugar: 6.9g; Sodium: 763mg; Fiber: 0.2g

283. Honey Garlic Chicken Wings

Servings: 4   Cooking Time: 1 Hour And 15 Minutes
Ingredients:
- 2 1/2 lb. chicken wings
- Poultry dry rub
- 4 tablespoons butter
- 3 cloves garlic, minced
- 1/2 cup hot sauce
- 1/4 cup honey

Directions:
Sprinkle chicken wings with dry rub.   Place on a baking pan.   Set the   wood pellet grill to 350 degrees F.   Preheat for 15 minutes while the lid is closed. Place the baking pan on the grill.   Cook for 50 minutes. Add butter to a pan over medium heat.   Sauté garlic for 3 minutes.   Stir in hot sauce and honey.   Cook for 5 minutes while stirring.   Coat the chicken wings with the mixture.   Grill for 10 more minutes.   Tips: You can make the sauce in advance to reduce preparation time.

284. Christmas Dinner Goose

Servings: 12   Cooking Time: 3 Hours
Ingredients:
- 1½ C. kosher salt
- 1 C. brown sugar
- 20 C. water
- 1 (12-lb.) whole goose, giblets removed
- 1 naval orange, cut into 6 wedges
- 1 large onion, cut into 8 wedges
- 2 bay leaves
- ¼ C. juniper berries, crushed
- 12 black peppercorns
- Salt and freshly ground black pepper, to taste
- 1 apple, cut into 6 wedges
- 2-3 fresh parsley sprigs

Directions:
Trim off any loose neck skin.   Then, trim the first two joints off the wings.   Wash the goose under cold running water and with paper towels, pat dry it.   With the tip of a paring knife, prick the goose all over the skin. In a large pitcher, dissolve kosher salt and brown sugar

in water.   Squeeze 3 orange wedges into brine.   Add goose, 4 onion wedges, bay leaves, juniper berries and peppercorns in brine and refrigerate for 24 hours.   Set the temperature of   Grill to 350 degrees F and preheat with closed lid for 15 minutes.   Remove the goose from brine and with paper towels, pat dry completely. Season the in and outside of goose with salt and black pepper evenly.   Stuff the cavity with apple wedges, herbs, remaining orange and onion wedges.   With kitchen strings, tie the legs together loosely.   Place the goose onto a rack arranged in a shallow roasting pan. Arrange the goose on grill and cook for about 1 hour. With a basting bulb, remove some of the fat from the pan and cook for about 1 hour.   Again, remove excess fat from the pan and cook for about ½-1 hour more. Remove goose from grill and place onto a cutting board for about 20 minutes before carving.   With a sharp knife, cut the goose into desired-sized pieces and serve.
Nutrition Info: Calories per serving: 907; Carbohydrates: 23.5g; Protein: 5.6g; Fat: 60.3g; Sugar: 19.9g; Sodium: 8000mg; Fiber: 1.1g

285. Smoked Drumsticks

Servings: 2 To 4   Cooking Time: 25 Minutes
Ingredients:
- 1 pound chicken drumsticks
- 2 tablespoons olive oil
- 1 batch Sweet and Spicy Cinnamon Rub

Directions:
Supply your smoker with wood pellets and follow the manufacturer's specific start-up procedure. Preheat the grill, with the lid closed, to 350°F.   Coat the drumsticks all over with olive oil and season with the rub. Using your hands, work the rub into the meat.   Place the drumsticks directly on the grill grate and smoke until their internal temperature reaches 170°F. Remove the drumsticks from the grill and serve immediately.

286. Chili Barbecue Chicken

Servings: 4   Cooking Time: 2 Hours And 10 Minutes
Ingredients:
- 1 tablespoon brown sugar
- 1 tablespoon lime zest
- 1 tablespoon chili powder
- 1/2 teaspoon ground cumin
- 1/2 tablespoon ground espresso
- Salt to taste
- 2 tablespoons olive oil
- 8 chicken legs
- 1/2 cup barbecue sauce

Directions:
Combine sugar, lime zest, chili powder, cumin, ground espresso and salt.   Drizzle the chicken legs with oil. Sprinkle sugar mixture all over the chicken.   Cover with foil and refrigerate for 5 hours.   Set the   wood pellet grill to 180 degrees F.   Preheat it for 15 minutes while the lid is closed.   Smoke the chicken legs for 1 hour.   Increase temperature to 350 degrees F.   Grill

the chicken legs for another 1 hour, flipping once. Brush the chicken with barbecue sauce and grill for another 10 minutes.   Tips: You can also add chili powder to the barbecue sauce.

287. Smoked Cornish Chicken In Wood Pellets

Servings: 6   Cooking Time: 1 Hour 10 Minutes
Ingredients:
- Cornish hens - 6
- Canola or avocado oil - 2-3 tbsp
- Spice mix - 6 tbsp

Directions:
Preheat your wood pellet grill to 275 degrees.   Rub the whole hen with oil and the spice mix. Use both of these ingredients liberally.   Place the breast area of the hen on the grill and smoke for 30 minutes.   Flip the hen, so the breast side is facing up. Increase the temperature to 400 degrees.   Cook until the temperature goes down to 165 degrees.   Pull it out and leave it for 10 minutes.   Serve warm with a side dish of your choice.
Nutrition Info: Carbohydrates: 1 g Protein: 57 g Fat: 50 g Sodium: 165 mg   Cholesterol: 337 mg

288. Rosemary Orange Chicken

Servings: 6   Cooking Time: 45 Minutes
Ingredients:
- 4 pounds chicken, backbone removed
- For the Marinade:
- 2 teaspoons salt
- 3 tablespoons chopped rosemary leaves
- 2 teaspoons Dijon mustard
- 1 orange, zested
- 1/4 cup olive oil
- ¼ cup of orange juice

Directions:
Prepare the chicken and for this, rinse the chicken, pat dry with paper towels and then place in a large baking dish.   Prepare the marinade and for this, take a medium bowl, place all of its ingredients in it and whisk until combined.   Cover chicken with the prepared marinade, cover with a plastic wrap, and then marinate for a minimum of 2 hours in the refrigerator, turning halfway.   When ready to cook, switch on the   grill, fill the grill hopper with flavored wood pellets, power the grill on by using the control panel, select 'smoke' on the temperature dial, or set the temperature to 350 degrees F and let it preheat for a minimum of 5 minutes. When the grill has preheated, open the lid, place chicken on the grill grate skin-side down, shut the grill and smoke for 45 minutes until well browned, and the internal temperature reaches 165 degrees F.   When done, transfer chicken to a cutting board, let it rest for 10 minutes, cut it into slices, and then serve.
Nutrition Info: Calories: 258 Cal ;Fat: 17.4 g ;Carbs: 5.2 g ;Protein: 19.3 g ;Fiber: 0.3 g

289. Wood-fired Chicken Breasts

Servings: 2 To 4   Cooking Time: 45 Minutes
Ingredients:
- 2 (1-pound) bone-in, skin-on chicken breasts
- 1 batch Chicken Rub

Directions:
Supply your smoker with wood pellets and follow the manufacturer's specific start-up procedure. Preheat the grill, with the lid closed, to 350°F.   Season the chicken breasts all over with the rub. Using your hands, work the rub into the meat.   Place the breasts directly on the grill grate and smoke until their internal temperature reaches 170°F. Remove the breasts from the grill and serve immediately.

290. Sheet Pan Chicken Fajitas

Servings: 10   Cooking Time: 10 Minutes
Ingredients:
- 2 lb chicken breast
- 1 onion, sliced
- 1 red bell pepper, seeded and sliced
- 1 orange-red bell pepper, seeded and sliced
- 1 tbsp salt
- 1/2 tbsp onion powder
- 1/2 tbsp granulated garlic
- 2 tbsp Spiceologist Chile Margarita Seasoning
- 2 tbsp oil

Directions:
Preheat the   to 450F and line a baking sheet with parchment paper.   In a mixing bowl, combine seasonings and oil then toss with the peppers and chicken.   Place the baking sheet in the   and let heat for 10 minutes with the lid closed.   Open the lid and place the veggies and the chicken in a single layer. Close the lid and cook for 10 minutes or until the chicken is no longer pink.   Serve with warm tortillas and top with your favorite toppings.

Nutrition Info: Calories 211, Total fat 6g, Saturated fat 1g, Total carbs 5g, Net carbs 4g Protein 29g, Sugars 4g, Fiber 1g, Sodium 360mg

291. Country Pork Roast

Servings: 8   Cooking Time: 3 Hours
Ingredients:
- 1 (28-ounce) jar or 2 (14.5-ounce) cans sauerkraut
- 3 Granny Smith apples, cored and chopped
- ¾ cup packed light brown sugar
- 3 tablespoons Greek seasoning
- 2 teaspoons dried basil leaves
- Extra-virgin olive oil, for rubbing
- 1 (2- to 2½-pound) pork loin roast

Directions:
Supply your smoker with wood pellets and follow the manufacturer's specific start-up procedure. Preheat, with the lid closed, to 250°F.   In a large bowl, stir together the sauerkraut, chopped apples, and brown sugar.   Spread the sauerkraut-apple mixture in the bottom of a 9-by-13-inch baking dish.   In a small bowl, mix together the Greek seasoning and dried basil for the rub.   Oil the pork roast and apply the rub, then place it fat-side up in the baking dish, on top of the sauerkraut. Transfer the baking dish to the grill, close the lid, and roast the pork for 3 hours, or until a meat thermometer inserted in the thickest part of the meat reads 160°F. Remove the pork roast from the baking dish and let rest for 5 minutes before slicing.   To serve, divide the sauerkraut-apple mixture among plates and top with the sliced pork.

292. Maple Baby Backs

Servings: 4 To 6   Cooking Time: 4 Hours
Ingredients:
- 2 (2- or 3-pound) racks baby back ribs
- 2 tablespoons yellow mustard
- 1 batch Sweet Brown Sugar Rub
- ½ cup plus 2 tablespoons maple syrup, divided
- 2 tablespoons light brown sugar
- 1 cup Pepsi or other non-diet cola
- ¼ cup The Ultimate BBQ Sauce

Directions:
Supply your smoker with wood pellets and follow the manufacturer's specific start-up procedure. Preheat the grill, with the lid closed, to 180°F.   Remove the membrane from the backside of the ribs. This can be done by cutting just through the membrane in an X pattern and working a paper towel between the membrane and the ribs to pull it off.   Coat the ribs on both sides with mustard and season them with the rub. Using your hands, work the rub into the meat.   Place the ribs directly on the grill grate and smoke for 3 hours. Remove the ribs from the grill and place them, bone-side up, on enough aluminum foil to wrap the ribs completely. Drizzle 2 tablespoons of maple syrup over the ribs and sprinkle them with 1 tablespoon of brown sugar. Flip the ribs and repeat the maple syrup and brown sugar

application on the meat side.   Increase the grill's temperature to 300°F.   Fold in three sides of the foil around the ribs and add the cola. Fold in the last side, completely enclosing the ribs and liquid. Return the ribs to the grill and cook for 30 to 45 minutes.   Remove the ribs from the grill and unwrap them from the foil.   In a small bowl, stir together the barbecue sauce and remaining 6 tablespoons of maple syrup. Use this to baste the ribs. Return the ribs to the grill, without the foil, and cook for 15 minutes to caramelize the sauce.   Cut into individual ribs and serve immediately.

293. Elegant Lamb Chops

Servings: 4   Cooking Time: 30 Minutes
Ingredients:
- 4 lamb shoulder chops
- 4 C. buttermilk
- 1 C. cold water
- ¼ C. kosher salt
- 2 tbsp. olive oil
- 1 tbsp. Texas-style rub

Directions:
In a large bowl, add buttermilk, water and salt and stir until salt is dissolved.   Add chops and coat with mixture evenly.   Refrigerate for at least 4 hours. Remove the chops from bowl and rinse under cold running water.   Coat the chops with olive oil and then sprinkle with rub evenly.   Set the temperature of Grill to 240 degrees F and preheat with closed lid for 15 minutes, using charcoal.   Arrange the chops onto grill and cook for about 25-30 minutes or until desired doneness.   Meanwhile, preheat the broiler of oven. Grease a broiler pan.   Remove the chops from grill and place onto the prepared broiler pan.   Transfer the broiler pan into the oven and broil for about 3-5 minutes or until browned.   Remove the chops from oven and serve hot.
Nutrition Info: Calories per serving: 414;
Carbohydrates: 11.7g; Protein: 5.6g; Fat: 22.7g; Sugar: 11.7g; Sodium: 7000mg; Fiber: 0g

294. Wood Pellet Grilled Shredded Pork Tacos

Servings: 8   Cooking Time: 7 Hours
Ingredients:
- 5 lb pork shoulder, bone-in
- Dry Rub
- 3 tbsp brown sugar
- 1 tbsp salt
- 1 tbsp garlic powder
- 1 tbsp paprika
- 1 tbsp onion powder
- 1/4 tbsp cumin
- 1 tbsp cayenne pepper

Directions:

Mix all the dry rub ingredients and rub on the pork shoulder. Preheat the grill to 275°F and cook the pork directly for 6 hours or until the internal temperature has reached 145°F. If you want to fall off the bone tender pork, then cook until the internal temperature is 190°F. Let rest for 10 minutes before serving. Enjoy

Nutrition Info: Calories 566, Total fat 41g, Saturated fat 15g, Total Carbs 4g, Net Carbs 4g, Protein 44g, Sugar 3g, Fiber 0g, Sodium: 659mg

295. Simply Delicious Tri Tip Roast

Servings: 8   Cooking Time: 35 Minutes
Ingredients:
- 1 tbsp. granulated onion
- 1 tbsp. granulated garlic
- Salt and freshly ground black pepper, to taste
- 1 (3-lb.) tri tip roast, trimmed

Directions:
In a bowl, add all ingredients except for roast and mix well. Coat the roast with spice mixture generously. Set aside at room temperature until grill heats. Set the temperature of Grill to 250 degrees F and preheat with closed lid for 15 minutes. Place the roast onto the grill and cook for about 25 minutes. Now, set the grill to 350-400 degrees F and preheat with closed lid for 15 minutes. and sear roast for about 3-5 minutes per side. Remove the roast from grill and place onto a cutting board for about 15-20 minutes before slicing. With a sharp knife, cut the roast into slices across the grain and serve.

Nutrition Info: Calories per serving: 313; Carbohydrates: 0.8g; Protein: 45.7g; Fat: 14.2g; Sugar: 0.3g; Sodium: 115mg; Fiber: 0.1g

296. Classic Pulled Pork

Servings: 8 To 12   Cooking Time: 16 To 20 Hours
Ingredients:
- 1 (6- to 8-pound) bone-in pork shoulder
- 2 tablespoons yellow mustard
- 1 batch Pork Rub

Directions:
Supply your smoker with wood pellets and follow the manufacturer's specific start-up procedure. Preheat the grill, with the lid closed, to 225°F. Coat the pork shoulder all over with mustard and season it with the rub. Using your hands, work the rub into the meat. Place the shoulder on the grill grate and smoke until its internal temperature reaches 195°F. Pull the shoulder from the grill and wrap it completely in aluminum foil or butcher paper. Place it in a cooler, cover the cooler, and let it rest for 1 or 2 hours. Remove the pork shoulder from the cooler and unwrap it. Remove the shoulder bone and pull the pork apart using just your fingers. Serve immediately as desired. Leftovers are encouraged.

297. Kalbi Beef Short Ribs

Servings: 6   Cooking Time: 6 Hours
Ingredients:
- 1/2 cup soy sauce
- 1/2 cup brown sugar
- 1/8 cup rice wine
- 2 tbsp minced garlic
- 1 tbsp sesame oil
- 1/8 cup onion, finely grated
- 2-1/2 pound beef short ribs, thinly sliced

Directions:
Mix soy sauce, sugar, rice wine, garlic, sesame oil and onion in a medium mixing bowl. Add the beef in the bowl and cover it in the marinade. Cover the bowl with a plastic wrap and refrigerate for 6 hours. Heat your to high and ensure the grill is well heated. Place on grill and close the lid ensuring you don't lose any heat. Cook for 4 minutes, flip, and cook for 4 more minutes on the other side. Remove the meat and serve with rice and veggies of choice. Enjoy.

Nutrition Info: Calories: 355 Cal Fat: 10 g Carbohydrates: 22 g   Protein: 28 g Fiber: 0 g

298. Wood Pellet Smoked Spicy Candied Bacon

Servings: 6   Cooking Time: 35 Minutes
Ingredients:
- 1 lb centre cut bacon
- 1/2 cup dark brown sugar
- 1/2 cup maple syrup
- 1 tbsp sriracha hot sauce
- 1/2 tbsp cayenne pepper

Directions:
In a mixing bowl, combine sugar, maple syrup, sriracha sauce, and cayenne pepper. Preheat the wood pellet grill to 300°F. Line a baking pan with parchment paper and lay the bacon on it in a single layer. Brush the bacon with the sugar mixture until well coated. Place the baking pan in the grill and cook for 20 minutes. Flip the bacon and cook for 15 more minutes. Remove the bacon from the grill and let cool for 10 minutes before removing from the baking pan and serving. Enjoy.

Nutrition Info: Calories 458, Total fat 14g, Saturated fat 10g, Total Carbs 37g, Net Carbs 37g, Protein 9g, Sugar 33g, Fiber 0g, Sodium: 565mg

299. Grilled Butter Basted Rib-eye

Servings: 4   Cooking Time: 20 Minutes
Ingredients:
- 2 rib-eye steaks, bone-in
- Slat to taste
- Pepper to taste
- 4 tbsp butter, unsalted

Directions:
Mix steak, salt, and pepper in a ziplock bag. Seal the bag and mix until the beef is well coated. Ensure you get as

much air as possible from the ziplock bag. Set the wood pellet grill temperature to high with closed lid for 15 minutes. Place a cast-iron into the grill. Place the steaks on the hottest spot of the grill and cook for 5 minutes with the lid closed. Open the lid and add butter to the skillet. When it's almost melted place the steak on the skillet with the grilled side up. Cook for 5 minutes while busting the meat with butter. Close the lid and cook until the internal temperature is 130°F. Remove the steak from skillet and let rest for 10 minutes before enjoying with the reserved butter.

Nutrition Info: Calories 745, Total fat 65g, Saturated fat 32g, Total Carbs 5g, Net Carbs 5g, Protein 35g, Sugar 0g, Fiber 0g

300. Lip-smackin' Pork Loin

Servings: 8   Cooking Time: 3 Hours
Ingredients:
- ¼ cup finely ground coffee
- ¼ cup paprika
- ¼ cup garlic powder
- 2 tablespoons chili powder
- 1 tablespoon packed light brown sugar
- 1 tablespoon ground allspice
- 1 tablespoon ground coriander
- 1 tablespoon freshly ground black pepper
- 2 teaspoons ground mustard
- 1½ teaspoons celery seeds
- 1 (1½- to 2-pound) pork loin roast

Directions:
Supply your smoker with wood pellets and follow the manufacturer's specific start-up procedure. Preheat, with the lid closed, to 250°F. In a small bowl, combine the ground coffee, paprika, garlic powder, chili powder, brown sugar, allspice, coriander, pepper, mustard, and celery seeds to create a rub, and generously apply it to the pork loin roast. Place the pork loin on the grill, fat-side up, close the lid, and roast for 3 hours, or until a meat thermometer inserted in the thickest part of the meat reads 160°F. Let the pork rest for 5 minutes before slicing and serving.

301. Naked St. Louis Ribs

Servings: 6-8   Cooking Time: 5-6 Hours
Ingredients:
- 3 St. Louis-style pork blacks
- 1 cup and 1 tablespoon of Yang's original dry lab or your favorite pork club

Directions:
Insert the spoon handle between the membrane and the rib bone and remove the membrane under the rib bone rack. Grasp the membrane with a paper towel and pull it down slowly from the rack to remove it. Rub both sides of the rib with a sufficient amount of friction. Use of wood pellet smokers and grills Configure a wood pellet smoker grill for indirect cooking and preheat to 225 ° F using hickory or apple pellets. If using Reblack, place the ribs on the grill grid rack. Otherwise,

you can use a Teflon-coated fiberglass mat or place the ribs directly on the grill. Slice rib bone at 225 ° F for 5-6 hours with hickory pellets until the internal temperature of the thickest part of the ick bone reaches 185 ° F to 190 ° F. Place ribs under loose foil tent for 10 minutes before carving and serving.

Nutrition Info: Calories: 320 Cal Fat: 26 g Carbohydrates: 0 g   Protein: 19 g Fiber: 0 g

302. Chinese Bbq Pork

Servings: 8   Cooking Time: 2 Hours
Ingredients:
- 2 pork tenderloins, silver skin removed
- For the Marinade:
- ½ teaspoon minced garlic
- 1 1/2 tablespoon brown sugar
- 1 teaspoon Chinese five-spice
- 1/4 cup honey
- 1 tablespoon Asian sesame oil
- 1/4 cup hoisin sauce
- 2 teaspoons red food coloring
- 1 tablespoon oyster sauce, optional
- 3 tablespoons soy sauce
- For the Five-Spice Sauce:
- 1/4 teaspoon Chinese five-spice
- 3 tablespoons brown sugar
- 1 teaspoon yellow mustard
- 1/4 cup ketchup

Directions:
Prepare the marinade and for this, take a small bowl, place all of its ingredients in it and whisk until combined. Take a large plastic bag, pour marinade in it, add pork tenderloin, seal the bag, turn it upside down to coat the pork and let it marinate for a minimum of 8 hours in the refrigerator. Switch on the grill, fill the grill hopper with maple-flavored wood pellets, power the grill on by using the control panel, select 'smoke' on the temperature dial, or set the temperature to 225 degrees F and let it preheat for a minimum of 5 minutes. Meanwhile, remove pork from the marinade, transfer marinade into a small saucepan, place it over medium-high heat and cook for 3 minutes, and then set aside until cooled. When the grill has preheated, open the lid, place pork on the grill grate, shut the grill and smoke for 2 hours, basting with the marinade halfway. Meanwhile, prepare the five-spice sauce and for this, take a small saucepan, place it over low heat, add all of its ingredients, stir until well combined and sugar has dissolved and cooked for 5 minutes until hot and thickened, set aside until required. When done, transfer pork to a dish, let rest for 15 minutes, and meanwhile, change the smoking temperature of the grill to 450 degrees F and let it preheat for a minimum of 10 minutes. Then return pork to the grill grate and cook for 3 minutes per side until slightly charred. Transfer pork to a dish, let rest for 5 minutes, and then serve with prepared five-spice sauce.

Nutrition Info: Calories: 280 Cal ;Fat: 8 g ;Carbs: 12 g ;Protein: 40 g ;Fiber: 0 g

303. Sweet And Hot Bbq Ribs

Servings: 4   Cooking Time: 5 Hours And 10 Minutes
Ingredients:
- 2 racks of pork ribs, bone-in, membrane removed
- 6 ounces pork and poultry rub
- 8 ounces apple juice
- 16 ounces sweet and heat BBQ sauce

Directions:
Sprinkle pork and poultry rub on all sides of pork ribs until evenly coated, rub well and marinate for a minimum of 30 minutes.   When ready to cook, switch on the   grill, fill the grill hopper with pecan flavored wood pellets, power the grill on by using the control panel, select 'smoke' on the temperature dial, or set the temperature to 225 degrees F and let it preheat for a minimum of 15 minutes.   When the grill has preheated, open the lid, place pork ribs on the grill grate bone-side down, shut the grill and smoke for 1 hour, spraying with 10 ounces of apple juice frequently.   Then wrap ribs in aluminum foil, pour in remaining 6 ounces of apple juice, and wrap tightly.   Return wrapped ribs onto the grill grate meat-side down, shut the grill and smoke for 3 to 4 hours until internal temperature reaches 203 degrees F. Remove wrapped ribs from the grill, uncover it and then brush well with the sauce.   Return pork ribs onto the grill grate and then grill for 10 minutes until glazed. When done, transfer ribs to a cutting board, let rest for 10 minutes, then cut it into slices and serve.
Nutrition Info: Calories: 250.8 Cal ;Fat: 16.3 g ;Carbs: 6.5 g ;Protein: 18.2 g ;Fiber: 0.2 g

304. Citrus-brined Pork Roast

Servings: 6   Cooking Time: 45 Minutes
Ingredients:
- ½ cup salt
- ¼ cup brown sugar
- 3 cloves of garlic, minced
- 2 dried bay leaves
- 6 peppercorns
- 1 lemon, juiced
- ½ teaspoon dried fennel seeds
- ½ teaspoon red pepper flakes
- ½ cup apple juice
- ½ cup orange juice
- 5 pounds pork loin
- 2 tablespoons extra virgin olive oil

Directions:
In a bowl, combine the salt, brown sugar, garlic, bay leaves, peppercorns, lemon juice, fennel seeds, pepper flakes, apple juice, and orange juice. Mix to form a paste rub.   Rub the mixture on to the pork loin and allow to marinate for at least 2 hours in the fridge. Add in the oil. When ready to cook, fire the   Grill to 300F. Use apple wood pellets when cooking. Close the lid and preheat for 15 minutes.   Place the seasoned pork loin on the grill grate and close the lid. Cook for 45 minutes. Make sure to flip the pork halfway through the cooking time.

Nutrition Info: Calories per serving: 869; Protein: 97.2g; Carbs: 15.2g; Fat: 43.9g Sugar: 13g

305. Pork Belly Burnt Ends

Servings: 8 To 10   Cooking Time: 6 Hours
Ingredients:
- 1 (3-pound) skinless pork belly (if not already skinned, use a sharp boning knife to remove the skin from the belly), cut into 1½- to 2-inch cubes
- 1 batch Sweet Brown Sugar Rub
- ½ cup honey
- 1 cup The Ultimate BBQ Sauce
- 2 tablespoons light brown sugar

Directions:
Supply your smoker with wood pellets and follow the manufacturer's specific start-up procedure. Preheat the grill, with the lid closed, to 250°F.   Generously season the pork belly cubes with the rub. Using your hands, work the rub into the meat.   Place the pork cubes directly on the grill grate and smoke until their internal temperature reaches 195°F.   Transfer the cubes from the grill to an aluminum pan. Add the honey, barbecue sauce, and brown sugar. Stir to combine and coat the pork.   Place the pan in the grill and smoke the pork for 1 hour, uncovered. Remove the pork from the grill and serve immediately.

306. Grilled Porterhouse Steak

Servings: 4   Cooking Time: 35 Minutes
Ingredients:
- 2 tablespoon Worcestershire sauce
- 2 teaspoon Dijon mustard
- 4 tablespoon butter
- Prime rib rub
- 2 porterhouse steaks

Directions:
Preheat your   wood pellet grill to 225 degrees F for 15 minutes while the lid is closed.   In a bowl, mix the Worcestershire sauce, mustard and butter.   Brush steaks with this mixture.   Sprinkle with the dry rub. Grill for 30 minutes, flipping once.   Increase temperature for 500 degrees F and grill for 2 minutes per side.   Tips: Choose steaks that are at least 1 ½ inch thick.

307. Reverse-seared Tri-tip

Servings: 4   Cooking Time: 2 To 3 Hours
Ingredients:
- 1½ pounds tri-tip roast
- 1 batch Espresso Brisket Rub

Directions:
Supply your   with wood pellets and follow the start-up procedure. Preheat the grill, with the lid closed, to 180°F. Season the tri-tip roast with the rub. Using your hands, work the rub into the meat.   Place the roast directly on the grill grate and smoke until its internal temperature

reaches 140°F.   Increase the grill's temperature to 450°F and continue to cook until the roast's internal temperature reaches 145°F. This same technique can be done over an open flame or in a cast-iron skillet with some butter.   Remove the tri-tip roast from the grill and let it rest 10 to 15 minutes, before slicing and serving.

308. Wood Pellet Grill Pork Crown Roast

Servings: 5   Cooking Time: 1 Hour
Ingredients:
- 13 ribs pork
- 1/4 cup favorite rub
- 1 cup apple juice
- 1 cup Apricot BBQ sauce

Directions:
Set the wood pellet temperature to 375°F to preheat for 15 minutes with the lid closed.   Meanwhile, season the pork with the rub then let sit for 30 minutes.   Wrap the tips of each crown roast with foil to prevent the borns from turning black.   Place the meat on the grill grate and cook for 90 minutes. Spray apple juice every 30 minutes.   When the meat has reached an internal temperature of 125°F remove the foils.   Spray the roast with apple juice again and let cook until the internal temperature has reached 135°F.   In the last 10 minutes of cooking, baste the roast with BBQ sauce.   Remove from the grill and wrap with foil. Let rest for 15 minutes before serving. Enjoy.
Nutrition Info: Calories 240, Total fat 16g, Saturated fat 6g, Total Carbs 0g, Net Carbs 0g, Protein 23g, Sugar 0g, Fiber 0g, Sodium: 50mg

309. Smoked Longhorn Cowboy Tri-tip

Servings: 7   Cooking Time: 4 Hours
Ingredients:
- 3 lb tri-tip roast
- 1/8 cup coffee, ground
- 1/4 cup   beef rub

Directions:
Preheat the grill to 180°F with the lid closed for 15 minutes.   Meanwhile, rub the roast with coffee and beef rub. Place the roast on the grill grate and smoke for 3 hours.   Remove the roast from the grill and double wrap it with foil. Increase the temperature to 275°F. Return the meat to the grill and let cook for 90 minutes or until the internal temperature reaches 135°F. Remove from the grill, unwrap it and let rest for 10 minutes before serving.   Enjoy.
Nutrition Info: Calories 245, Total fat 14g, Saturated fat 4g, Total Carbs 0g, Net Carbs 0g, Protein 23g, Sugar 0g, Fiber 0g, Sodium: 80mg

310. Brown Sugar Lamb Chops

Servings: 4   Cooking Time: 10-15 Minutes
Ingredients:
- Pepper

- One t. garlic powder
- Salt
- Two t. tarragon
- One t. cinnamon
- ¼ c. brown sugar
- 4 lamb chops
- Two t. ginger

Directions:
Combine the salt, garlic powder, pepper, cinnamon, tarragon, ginger, and sugar. Coat the lamb chops in the mixture and chill for two hours.   Add wood pellets to your smoker and follow your cooker's startup procedure. Preheat your smoker, with your lid closed, until it reaches 450. Place the chops on the grill, cover, and smoke for 10-15 minutes per side. Serve.
Nutrition Info: Calories: 210 Cal Fat: 11 g Carbohydrates: 3 g   Protein: 25 g Fiber: 1 g

311. Roasted Pork With Balsamic Strawberry Sauce

Servings: 3   Cooking Time: 35 Minutes
Ingredients:
- 2 lb pork tenderloin
- Salt and pepper to taste
- 2 tbsp rosemary, dried
- 2 tbsp olive oil
- 12 strawberries, fresh
- 1 cup balsamic vinegar
- 4 tbsp sugar

Directions:
Set the wood pellet grill to 350°F and preheat for 15 minutes with a closed lid.   Meanwhile, rinse the pork and pat it dry. Season with salt, pepper, and rosemary. In an oven skillet, heat oil until smoking. Add the pork and sear on all sides until golden brown.   Set the skillet in the grill and cook for 20 minutes or until the meat is no longer pink and the internal temperature is 150°F. Remove the pork from the grill and let rest for 10 minutes. Add berries to the skillet and sear over the stovetop for a minute. Remove the strawberries from the skillet. Add vinegar in the same skillet and scrape any browned bits from the skillet bottom. Bring it to boil then reduce heat to low. Stir in sugar and cook until it has reduced by half.   Slice the meat and place the strawberries on top then drizzle vinegar sauce. Enjoy.
Nutrition Info: Calories 244, Total fat 9g, Saturated fat 3g, Total Carbs 15g, Net Carbs 13g, Protein 25g, Sugar 12g, Fiber 2g, Sodium: 159mg

312. Grilled Lamb Burgers

Servings: 5   Cooking Time: 15 Minutes
Ingredients:
- 1 1/4 pounds of ground lamb.
- 1 egg.
- 1 teaspoon of dried oregano.
- 1 teaspoon of dry sherry.
- 1 teaspoon of white wine vinegar.
- 4 minced cloves of garlic.

- Red pepper
- 1/2 cup of chopped green onions.
- 1 tablespoon of chopped mint.
- 2 tablespoons of chopped cilantro.
- 2 tablespoons of dry bread crumbs.
- 1/8 teaspoon of salt to taste.
- 1/4 teaspoon of ground black pepper to taste.
- 5 hamburger buns.

Directions:
Preheat a Wood Pellet Smoker or Grill to 350-450 degrees F then grease it grates. Using a large mixing bowl, add in all the ingredients on the list aside from the buns then mix properly to combine with clean hands. Make about five patties out of the mixture .then set aside.   Place the lamb patties on the preheated grill and cook for about seven to nine minutes turning only once until an inserted thermometer reads 160 degrees F. Serve the lamb burgers on the hamburger, add your favorite toppings and enjoy.
Nutrition Info: Calories: 376 Cal Fat: 18.5 g Carbohydrates: 25.4 g Protein: 25.5 g Fiber: 1.6 g

313. Wood Pellet Smoked Lamb Shoulder

Servings: 7   Cooking Time: 1hour 30 Minutes;
Ingredients:
- For Smoked Lamb Shoulder
- 5 lb lamb shoulder, boneless and excess fat trimmed
- 2 tbsp kosher salt
- 2 tbsp black pepper
- 1 tbsp rosemary, dried
- The Injection
- 1 cup apple cider vinegar
- The Spritz
- 1 cup apple cider vinegar
- 1 cup apple juice

Directions:
Preheat the wood pellet smoker with a water pan to 225 F.   Rinse the lamb in cold water then pat it dry with a paper towel. Inject vinegar to the lamb.   Pat the lamb dry again and rub with oil, salt black pepper and rosemary. Tie with kitchen twine.   Smoke uncovered for 1 hour then spritz after every 15 minutes until the internal temperature reaches 195 F.   Remove the lamb from the grill and place it on a platter. Let cool before shredding it and enjoying it with your favorite side.
Nutrition Info: Calories 243, Total fat 19g, Saturated fat 8g, Total Carbs 0g, Net Carbs 0g, Protein 17g, Sugar 0g, Fiber 1g, Sodium: 63mg, Potassium 234mg

314. Easy-to-prepare Lamb Chops

Servings: 6   Cooking Time: 12 Minutes
Ingredients:
- 6 (6-oz.) lamb chops
- 3 tbsp. olive oil
- Salt and freshly ground black pepper, to taste

Directions:

Set the temperature of   Grill to 450 degrees F and preheat with closed lid for 15 minutes.   Coat the lamb chops with oil and then, season with salt and black pepper evenly.   Arrange the chops onto the grill and cook for about 4-6 minutes per side.   Remove the chops from grill and serve hot.
Nutrition Info: Calories per serving: 376; Carbohydrates: 0g; Protein: 47.8g; Fat: 19.5g; Sugar: 0g; Sodium: 156mg; Fiber: 0g

315. Smoked Lamb Chops

Servings: 4   Cooking Time: 50 Minutes
Ingredients:
- 1 rack lamb
- 2 tbsp rosemary, fresh
- 2 tbsp sage, fresh
- 1 tbsp thyme, fresh
- 2 garlic cloves, roughly chopped
- 2 tbsp shallots, roughly chopped
- 1/2 tbsp salt
- 1/2 tbsp ground pepper
- 1/4 cup olive oil
- 1 tbsp honey

Directions:
Preheat the   to 225F   Trim any excess fat and silver skin from the lamb.   Combine the rest of the ingredients in the food processor and generously rub the lamb with the seasoning.   Place the seasoned lamb on the   and cook for 45 minutes or until the internal temperature reaches 120F.   Sear the lamb on the   for 2 minutes per side or until the internal temperature reaches 125F for medium-rare or 145F for medium. Let rest for 5 minutes before slicing it. Enjoy
Nutrition Info: Calories 916, Total fat 78.3g, Saturated fat 33.9g, Total carbs 2.7g, Net carbs 2.2g Protein 47g, Sugars 0.1g, Fiber 0.5g, Sodium 1324mmg

316. Wet-rubbed St. Louis Ribs

Servings: 3   Cooking Time: 4 Hours
Ingredients:
- 1/2 cup brown sugar
- 1 tbsp cumin, ground
- 1 tbsp Ancho Chile powder
- 1 tbsp smoked paprika
- 1 tbsp garlic salt
- 3 tbsp balsamic vinegar
- 1 Rack St. Louis style ribs
- 2 cup apple juice

Directions:
Add all the ingredients except ribs in a mixing bowl and mix until well mixed. Place the rub on both sides of the ribs and let sit for 10 minutes.   Set the wood pellet temperature to 180°F and preheat for 15 minutes. Smoke the ribs for 2 hours.   Increase the temperature to 250°F and wrap the ribs and apple juice with foil or in tinfoil.   Place back the pork and cook for an additional 2 hours.   Remove from the grill and let rest for 10 minutes before serving. Enjoy.

Nutrition Info: Calories 210, Total fat 13g, Saturated fat 4g, Total Carbs 0g, Net Carbs 0g, Protein 24g, Sugar 0g, Fiber 0g, Sodium: 85mg

317. Lamb Shank

Servings: 6   Cooking Time: 4 Hours
Ingredients:
- 8-ounce red wine
- 2-ounce whiskey
- 2 tablespoons minced fresh rosemary
- 1 tablespoon minced garlic
- Black pepper
- 6 (1¼-pound) lamb shanks

Directions:
In a bowl, add all ingredients except lamb shank and mix till well combined.   In a large resealable bag, add marinade and lamb shank.   Seal the bag and shake to coat completely.   Refrigerate for about 24 hours. Preheat the pallet grill to 225 degrees F.   Arrange the leg of lamb in pallet grill and cook for about 4 hours.
Nutrition Info: Calories: 1507 Cal Fat: 62 g Carbohydrates: 68.7 g   Protein:163.3 g Fiber: 6 g

318. Grilled Butter Basted Steak

Servings: 2   Cooking Time: 40 Minutes
Ingredients:
- 2 steaks, each about 16 ounces, 1 ½-inch thick
- Rib rub as needed
- 2 teaspoon Dijon mustard
- 2 tablespoons Worcestershire sauce
- 4 tablespoons butter, unsalted, melted

Directions:
Switch on the   grill, fill the grill hopper with hickory wood pellets, power the grill on by using the control panel, select 'smoke' on the temperature dial, or set the temperature to 225 degrees F and let it preheat for a minimum of 15 minutes.   Meanwhile, take a small bowl, place mustard, Worcestershire sauce, and butter in it and stir until well combined.   Brush the mixture on both sides of steaks and then season with rib rub. When the grill has preheated, open the lid, place food on the grill grate, shut the grill, and smoke for 30 minutes. When done, transfer steaks to a dish, let rest for 15 minutes, and meanwhile, change the smoking temperature of the grill to 450 degrees F and let it preheat for a minimum of 10 minutes.   Then return steaks to the grill grate and cook for 3 minutes per side until the internal temperature reaches 140 degrees F. Transfer steaks to a dish, let rest for 5 minutes and then serve.
Nutrition Info: Calories: 409.8 Cal ;Fat: 30.8 g ;Carbs: 3.1 g ;Protein: 29.7 g ;Fiber: 0.4 g

319. Bacon-wrapped Sausages In Brown Sugar

Servings: 8   Cooking Time: 30 Minutes

Ingredients:
- 1 pound bacon strips, halved
- 14 ounces cocktail sausages
- ½ cup brown sugar

Directions:
Place bacon strips on clean working space, roll them by using a rolling pin, and then wrap a sausage with a bacon strip, securing with a toothpick.   Place wrapped sausage in a casserole dish, repeat with the other sausages, place them into the casserole dish in a single layer, cover with sugar and then let them sit for 30 minutes in the refrigerator.   When ready to cook, switch on the   grill, fill the grill hopper with apple-flavored wood pellets, power the grill on by using the control panel, select 'smoke' on the temperature dial, or set the temperature to 350 degrees F and let it preheat for a minimum of 15 minutes.   Meanwhile, remove the casserole dish from the refrigerator and then arrange sausage on a cookie sheet lined with parchment paper. When the grill has preheated, open the lid, place cookie sheet on the grill grate, shut the grill and smoke for 30 minutes.   When done, transfer sausages to a dish and then serve.
Nutrition Info: Calories: 270 Cal ;Fat: 27 g ;Carbs: 18 g ;Protein: 9 g ;Fiber: 2 g

320. Grill A Burger Without Flipping Them

Servings: 6   Cooking Time: 45-50 Minutes
Ingredients:
- 1 Ground Beef Patties
- Beef Rub
- Cheese
- Pretzel buns

Directions:
Start with cold but not frozen patties and sprinkle on the Beef Rub and massage into both side of the patty. Preheat grill to 250 degrees and cook for 45 minutes Add cheese and other topic varieties of your liking Close the grill back up and let them finish for another 10 minutes before removing
Nutrition Info: Calories: 696 Cal Fat: 54 g Carbohydrates: 11 g   Protein: 38 g Fiber: 0 g

321. Peppered Beef Tenderloin

Servings: 6   Cooking Time: 1 Hour And 15 Minutes
Ingredients:
- 2 1/2 lb center cut beef tenderloin, trimmed and tied if uneven
- 2 tbsp unsalted butter, room temperature
- 6 tbsp peppercorns, mixed colors
- 1 tbsp kosher salt
- 1 cup parsley, chopped
- Horseradish sauce, on the side
- 4 tbsp Dijon mustard

Directions:
Coarsely grind peppercorn mixture into a bowl. Add parsley, mustard, butter, and salt. Mix until thoroughly combined   Rub spiced butter mixture generously and

thoroughly on all sides of the tenderloin. Coat completely and roll tenderloin in bowl if necessary to soak up as much seasoning as possible.   Preheat pellet grill to 450°F4. Place tenderloin on an elevated rack (important) and roast. Use a probe meat thermometer to measure internal temperature. Cook until the center of the tenderloin reaches a temperature of 130°F. This typically takes 30-45 minutes but could be more or less depending on the size of your tenderloin   Once tenderloin reaches desired doneness, remove from grill and allow to rest for at least 15 minutes6. Move tenderloin to a cutting board and slice. Try to catch as many juices as possible. Garnish with additional parsley

322. Real Treat Chuck Roast

Servings: 8   Cooking Time: 4½ Hours
Ingredients:
- 2 tbsp. onion powder
- 2 tbsp. garlic powder
- 1 tbsp. red chili powder
- 1 tbsp. cayenne pepper
- Salt and freshly ground black pepper, to taste
- 1 (3 lb.) beef chuck roast
- 16 fluid oz. warm beef broth

Directions:
Set the temperature of   Grill to 250 degrees F and preheat with closed lid for 15 minutes.   In a bowl, mix together spices, salt and black pepper.   Rub the chuck roast with spice mixture evenly.   Place the rump roast onto the grill and cook for about 1½ hours per side. Now, arrange chuck roast in a steaming pan with beef broth.   With a piece of foil, cover the pan and cook for about 2-3 hours.   Remove the chuck roast from grill and place onto a cutting board for about 20 minutes before slicing.   With a sharp knife, cut the chuck roast into desired-sized slices and serve.

Nutrition Info: Calories per serving: 645; Carbohydrates: 4.2g; Protein: 46.4g; Fat: 48g; Sugar: 1.4g; Sodium: 329mg; Fiber: 1g

323. Cheeseburger Hand Pies

Servings: 4   Cooking Time: 10 Minutes
Ingredients:
- ½ pound lean ground beef
- 1 tablespoon minced onion
- 1 tablespoon steak seasoning
- 1 cup shredded Monterey Jack and Colby cheese blend
- 8 slices white American cheese, divided
- 2 (14-ounce) refrigerated prepared pizza dough sheets, divided
- 2 eggs, beaten with 2 tablespoons water (egg wash), divided
- 24 hamburger dill pickle chips
- 2 tablespoons sesame seeds
- 6 slices tomato, for garnish
- Ketchup and mustard, for serving

Directions:

Supply your smoker with wood pellets and follow the manufacturer's specific start-up procedure. Preheat, with the lid closed, to 325°F.   On your stove top, in a medium sauté pan over medium-high heat, brown the ground beef for 4 to 5 minutes, or until cooked through. Add the minced onion and steak seasoning.   Toss in the shredded cheese blend and 2 slices of American cheese, and stir until melted and fully incorporated. Remove the cheeseburger mixture from the heat and set aside.   Make sure the dough is well chilled for easier handling. Working quickly, roll out one prepared pizza crust on parchment paper and brush with half of the egg wash.   Arrange the remaining 6 slices of American cheese on the dough to outline 6 hand pies.   Top each cheese slice with ¼ cup of the cheeseburger mixture, spreading slightly inside the imaginary lines of the hand pies.   Place 4 pickle slices on top of the filling for each pie.   Top the whole thing with the other prepared pizza crust and cut between the cheese slices to create 6 hand pies.   Using kitchen scissors, cut the parchment to further separate the pies, but leave them on the paper. 1Using a fork dipped in egg wash, seal the edges of the pies on all sides. Baste the tops of the pies with the remaining egg wash and sprinkle with the sesame seeds. 1Remove the pies from the parchment paper and gently place on the grill grate. Close the lid and smoke for 5 minutes, then carefully flip and smoke with the lid closed for 5 more minutes, or until browned.   1Top with the sliced tomato and serve with ketchup and mustard.

324. Smoked Pork Sausages

Servings: 6   Cooking Time: 1 Hour
Ingredients:
- 3 pounds ground pork
- ½ tablespoon ground mustard
- 1 tablespoon onion powder
- 1 tablespoon garlic powder
- 1 teaspoon pink curing salt
- 1 teaspoon salt
- 1 teaspoon black pepper
- ¼ cup ice water
- Hog casings, soaked and rinsed in cold water

Directions:
Mix all ingredients except for the hog casings in a bowl. Using your hands, mix until all ingredients are well-combined.   Using a sausage stuffer, stuff the hog casings with the pork mixture.   Measure 4 inches of the stuffed hog casing and twist to form into a sausage. Repeat the process until you create sausage links. When ready to cook, fire the   Grill to 225F. Use apple wood pellets when cooking the ribs. Close the lid and preheat for 15 minutes.   Place the sausage links on the grill grate and cook for 1 hour or until the internal temperature of the sausage reads at 155F.   Allow to rest before slicing.

Nutrition Info: Calories per serving: 688; Protein: 58.9g; Carbs: 2.7g; Fat: 47.3g Sugar: 0.2g

325. Smoked Ham Recipe

Servings: 4   Cooking Time: 12-15 Minutes
Ingredients:
- 4 ounces of smoked ham, scored
- 1/2 cup of butter
- 2 tablespoons of brown sugar
- 1tablespoon of honey
- 2tablespoons of pineapple cane syrup

Directions:
Place the grill rack inside and pour a cup of water in it, then close the unit.   Let it preheat for 20 minutes at high.   Meanwhile, melt butter in a cooking pot and add two tablespoons of brown sugar.   Melt it down and add a tablespoon of honey and pineapple cane syrup. Mix well, and let it get simmer until thickened.   Turn off the grill and open the unit.   Then brush the ham with glaze.   Close the unit and cook for 7 minutes. After 5 minutes, open the unit by turning it off and glazed the ham again.   Cook for remaining 2 minutes Sprinkle the ham with any favorite spice blend.   Slice and serve.
Nutrition Info: Calories: 291 Total Fat: 25.5gSaturated Fat: 15.4gCholesterol: 77mg Sodium: 535mg Total Carbohydrate: 12g Dietary Fiber 0.5g Total Sugars: 10.7g Protein: 5g

326. Crown Rack Of Lamb

Servings: 6   Cooking Time: 30 Minutes
Ingredients:
- 2 racks of lamb, frenched
- 1 tbsp garlic, crushed
- 1 tbsp rosemary, finely chopped
- 1/4 cup olive oil
- 2 feet twine

Directions:
Rinse the racks with cold water then pat them dry with a paper towel.   Lay the racks on a flat board then score between each bone, about 1/4 inch down.   In a mixing bowl, mix garlic, rosemary, and oil then generously brush on the lamb.   Take each lamb rack and bend it into a semicircle forming a crown-like shape.   Use the twine to wrap the racks about 4 times starting from the base to the top. Make sure you tie the twine tightly to keep the racks together.   Preheat the wood pellet to 400-450 F then place the lamb racks on a baking dish. Plac ethe baing dish on the pellet grill.   Cook for 10 minutes then reduce temperature to 300 F. cook for 20 more minutes or until the internal temperature reaches 130 F.   Remove the lamb rack from the wood pellet and let rest for 15 minutes.   Serve when hot with veggies and potatoes. Enjoy.
Nutrition Info: Calories 390, Total fat 35g, Saturated fat 15g, Total Carbs 0g, Net Carbs 0g, Protein 17g, Sugar 0g, Fiber 0g, Sodium: 65mg.

327. Grilled Lamb Sandwiches

Servings: 6   Cooking Time: 50 Minutes

Ingredients:
- 1 (4 pounds) boneless lamb.
- 1 cup of raspberry vinegar.
- 2 tablespoons of olive oil.
- 1 tablespoon of chopped fresh thyme.
- 2 pressed garlic cloves.
- 1/4 teaspoon of salt to taste.
- 1/4 teaspoon of ground pepper.
- Sliced bread.

Directions:
Using a large mixing bowl, add in the raspberry vinegar, oil, and thyme then mix properly to combine. Add in the lamb, toss to combine then let it sit in the refrigerator for about eight hours or overnight.   Next, discard the marinade the season the lamb with salt and pepper to taste. Preheat a Wood Pellet Smoker and grill to 400-500 degrees F, add in the seasoned lamb and grill for about thirty to forty minutes until it attains a temperature of 150 degrees F. Once cooked, let the lamb cool for a few minutes, slice as desired then serve on the bread with your favorite topping.
Nutrition Info: Calories: 407 Cal Fat: 23 g Carbohydrates: 26 g   Protein: 72 g Fiber: 2.3 g

328. Smoked Roast Beef

Servings: 5 To 8   Cooking Time: 12 To 14 Hours
Ingredients:
- 1 (4-pound) top round roast
- 1 batch Espresso Brisket Rub
- 1 tablespoon butter

Directions:
Supply your   with wood pellets and follow the start-up procedure. Preheat the grill, with the lid closed, to 180°F. Season the top round roast with the rub. Using your hands, work the rub into the meat.   Place the roast directly on the grill grate and smoke until its internal temperature reaches 140°F. Remove the roast from the grill.   Place a cast-iron skillet on the grill grate and increase the grill's temperature to 450°F. Place the roast in the skillet, add the butter, and cook until its internal temperature reaches 145°F, flipping once after about 3 minutes.   Remove the roast from the grill and let it rest for 10 to 15 minutes, before slicing and serving.

329. Aromatic Herbed Rack Of Lamb

Servings: 3   Cooking Time: 2 Hours
Ingredients:
- 2 tbsp. fresh sage
- 2 tbsp. fresh rosemary
- 2 tbsp. fresh thyme
- 2 garlic cloves, peeled
- 1 tbsp. honey
- Salt and freshly ground black pepper, to taste
- ¼ C. olive oil
- 1 (1½-lb.) rack of lamb, trimmed

Directions:
In a food processor, add all ingredients except for oil and rack of lamb rack and pulse until well combined.

While motor is running, slowly add oil and pulse until a smooth paste is formed.   Coat the rib rack with paste generously and refrigerate for about 2 hours.   Set the temperature of Grill to 225 degrees F and preheat with closed lid for 15 minutes.   Arrange the rack of lamb onto the grill and cook for about 2 hours.   Remove the rack of lamb from grill and place onto a cutting board for about 10-15 minutes before slicing.   With a sharp knife, cut the rack into individual ribs and serve.

Nutrition Info: Calories per serving: 566; Carbohydrates: 9.8g; Protein: 46.7g; Fat: 33.5g; Sugar: 5.8g; Sodium: 214mg; Fiber: 2.2g

330. Grill Marinated Steak

Servings: 2   Cooking Time: 8 Minutes
Ingredients:
- 12 ounces of steak
- Steak Marinade Ingredients:
- 1/4 cup canola oil
- 3 cloves garlic, minced
- 1/4 teaspoon dried rosemary
- 1/3 teaspoon dried oregano
- 1/4 teaspoon dried thyme
- 1/4 teaspoon dried basil
- Salt and black pepper, to taste

Directions:
Mix all the marinade Ingredients in a zip lock pack and put steak inside the zip lock pack   Marinate the steak in marinating liquid for 20 minutes.   Insert grill grate inside the grill and close the hood.   Preheat it for 10 minutes at Max.   Once preheated, the add food signal comes on display.   Open the grill and put the meat inside the grill.   Close the lid of the unit and grill for 4-5 minutes.   Open and flip the steak and close the unit. Grill for 4 more minutes.   Once done, serve and enjoy.

Nutrition Info: Calories: 588 Total Fat: 35.8g46% Saturated Fat: 5g25% Cholesterol: 153mg51% Sodium: 78mg3% Total Carbohydrate: 1.9g1% Dietary Fiber 0.3g1% Total Sugars: 0.1g Protein: 61.8g

331. Bison Tomahawk Steak

Servings: 4   Cooking Time: 12 Minutes
Ingredients:
- 2 ½ whole bone-in buffalo rib-eye steak
- 2 teaspoons cherrywood smoked salt
- 1 ½ tablespoons black pepper

Directions:
Fire the   Grill to 450F. Use desired wood pellets when cooking. Close the lid and preheat for 15 minutes. Season the rib-eye steak with salt and pepper to taste. Place the steak directly on the grill grate. Grill for 6 minutes on each side or until the internal temperature reaches 140F.   Remove from the grill and allow to rest before slicing.

Nutrition Info: Calories per serving: 751; Protein: 51.6g; Carbs: 1.7g; Fat: 60.1g; Sugar: 0.02g

332. Pulled Pork

Servings: 12   Cooking Time: 9 Hours
Ingredients:
- 9 pounds pork shoulder, bone-in, fat trimmed
- Game rub as needed and more as required
- 2cups apple cider

Directions:
Switch on the   grill, fill the grill hopper with apple-flavored wood pellets, power the grill on by using the control panel, select 'smoke' on the temperature dial, or set the temperature to 250 degrees F and let it preheat for a minimum of 15 minutes.   Meanwhile, prepare the pork shoulder, and for this, season it generously with game rub until well coated.   When the grill has preheated, open the lid, place pork should on the grill grate fat-side up, shut the grill and smoke for 5 hours, and then remove pork from the grill.   Take a large baking sheet, line it with 4 large aluminum foil pieces to wrap pork, place pork in the center, bring up the foil's sides, pour in apple cider, and then wrap tightly.   Transfer baking sheet containing wrapped pork on the grill grate and then cook for 4 hours until the internal temperature reaches 204 degrees F.   When done, remove the baking sheet from the grill, let it rest for 45 minutes, then uncover it, place the pork into a large dish and drain excess liquid into a bowl.   Shred pork by using two forks, remove and discard excess fat and bone, then drizzle with reserved liquid and season with some game rub.   Serve straight away.

Nutrition Info: Calories: 220.1 Cal Fat: 15 g Carbs: 1 g Protein: 20 g Fiber: 0 g

333. Spicy Chinese Cumin Lamb Skewers

Servings: 10   Cooking Time: 6 Minutes
Ingredients:
- 1lb lamb shoulder, cut into 1/2 inch pieces
- 10 skewers
- 2 tbsp ground cumin
- 2 tbsp red pepper flakes
- 1 tbsp salt

Directions:
Thread the lamb pieces onto skewers.   Preheat the wood pellet grill to medium heat and lightly oil the grill grate.   Place the skewers on the grill grate and cook while turning occasionally. Sprinkle cumin, pepper flakes, and salt every time you turn the skewer.   Cook for 6 minutes or until nicely browned.   Serve and enjoy.

Nutrition Info: Calories 77, Total fat 5.2g, Saturated fat 2g, Total Carbs 1.6g, Net Carbs 1g, Protein 6.3g, Sugar0g, Fiber 0.6g, Sodium: 715mg, Potassium 110mg

334. Apple-smoked Pork Tenderloin

Servings: 4 To 6   Cooking Time: 4 To 5 Hours
Ingredients:
- 2 (1-pound) pork tenderloins
- 1 batch Pork Rub

Directions:

Supply your smoker with wood pellets and follow the manufacturer's specific start-up procedure. Preheat the grill, with the lid closed, to 180°F.   Generously season the tenderloins with the rub. Using your hands, work the rub into the meat.   Place the tenderloins directly on the grill grate and smoke for 4 or 5 hours, until their internal temperature reaches 145°F.   Remove the tenderloins from the grill and let them rest for 5 to 10 minutes before thinly slicing and serving.

335. Smoked Sausages

Servings: 4   Cooking Time: 3 Hours
Ingredients:
- 3 pounds ground pork
- 1 tablespoon onion powder
- 1 tablespoon garlic powder
- 1 teaspoon curing salt
- 4 teaspoon black pepper
- 1/2 tablespoon salt
- 1/2 tablespoon ground mustard
- Hog casings, soaked
- 1/2 cup ice water

Directions:
Switch on the   grill, fill the grill hopper with flavored wood pellets, power the grill on by using the control panel, select 'smoke' on the temperature dial, or set the temperature to 225 degrees F and let it preheat for a minimum of 15 minutes.   Meanwhile, take a medium bowl, place all the ingredients in it except for water and hog casings, and stir until well mixed.   Pour in water, stir until incorporated, place the mixture in a sausage stuffer, then stuff the hog casings and tie the link to the desired length.   When the grill has preheated, open the lid, place the sausage links on the grill grate, shut the grill, and smoke for 2 to 3 hours until the internal temperature reaches 155 degrees F.   When done, transfer sausages to a dish, let them rest for 5 minutes, then slice and serve.
Nutrition Info: Calories: 230 Cal ;Fat: 22 g ;Carbs: 2 g ;Protein: 14 g ;Fiber: 0 g

336. Slow Roasted Shawarma

Servings: 6-8   Cooking Time: 4 Hours 55 Minutes
Ingredients:
- Top sirloin - 5.5 lbs
- Lamb fat - 4.5 lbs
- Boneless, skinless chicken thighs- 5.5 lbs
- Pita bread
- rub - 4 tbsp
- Double skewer - 1
- Large yellow onions - 2
- Variety of topping options such as tomatoes, cucumbers, pickles, tahini, Israeli salad, fries, etc.
- Cast iron griddle

Directions:
Assemble the stack of shawarma the night before you wish to cook it.   Slice all the meat and fat into ½-inch slices. Place them into 3 bowls. If you partially freeze them, it will be much easier to slice them.   Season the

bowl with the rub, massaging it thoroughly into the meat. Place half a yellow onion on the bottom of the skewers to ensure a firm base. Add 2 layers at a time from each bowl. Try to make the entire stack symmetrical. Place the other 2 onions on top. Wrap them in plastic wrap and refrigerate overnight.   When the meat is ready to cook, preheat the pellet grill for about 15 minutes with the lid closed at a temperature of 275 degrees Fahrenheit. Lay the shawarma directly on the grill grate and cook it for at least 3-4 hours. Rotate the skewers at least once. Remove them from the grill and increase its temperature to 445 degrees Fahrenheit. When the grill is preheating, place a cast iron griddle directly on the grill grate and brush it with some olive oil.   Once the griddle is hot enough, place the shawarma directly on the cast iron. Sear it on each side for 5-10 minutes. Remove it from the grill and slice off the edges. Repeat the process with the remaining shawarma.   Serve in pita bread and favorite toppings, such as tomatoes, cucumbers, Israeli salad, fries, pickles, or tahini. Enjoy!
Nutrition Info: Carbohydrates: 4.6 g Protein: 30.3 g Fat: 26.3 g Sodium: 318.7 mg Cholesterol: 125.5 mg

337. Blackened Pork Chops

Servings: 6   Cooking Time: 20 Minutes
Ingredients:
- 6 pork chops
- 1/4 cup blackening seasoning
- Salt and pepper

Directions:
Preheat your   to 375F.   Generously season the pork chops with the blackening seasoning, salt, and pepper. Place the chops on the   grill and cook for 8 minutes on one side then flip.   Cook until the internal temperature reaches 1420F.   Let the pork chops rest for 10 minutes before slicing and serving.
Nutrition Info: Calories 333, Total fat 18g, Saturated fat 6g, Total carbs 1g, Net carbs 0g Protein 40g, Sugars 0g, Fiber 1g, Sodium 3175mg

338. Prime Rib Roast

Servings: 8   Cooking Time: 4 Hours And 30 Minutes
Ingredients:
- 1 prime rib roast, containing 5 to 7 bones
- Rib rub as needed

Directions:
Season rib roast with rib rub until well coated, place it in a large plastic bag, seal it and let it marinate for a minimum of 24 hours in the refrigerator.   When ready to cook, switch on the   grill, fill the grill hopper with cherry flavored wood pellets, power the grill on by using the control panel, select 'smoke' on the temperature dial, or set the temperature to 225 degrees F and let it preheat for a minimum of 15 minutes.   When the grill has preheated, open the lid, place rib roast on the grill grate fat-side up, change the smoking temperature to 425 degrees F, shut the grill, and smoke for 30 minutes. Then change the smoking temperature to 325 degrees F

and continue cooking for 3 to 4 hours until roast has cooked to the desired level, rare at 120 degrees F, medium rare at 130 degrees F, medium at 140 degrees F, and well done at 150 degrees F.   When done, transfer roast rib to a cutting board, let it rest for 15 minutes, then cut it into slices and serve.
Nutrition Info: Calories: 248 Cal ;Fat: 21.2 g ;Carbs: 0 g ;Protein: 28 g ;Fiber: 0 g

339. Crown Rack Of Lamb

Servings: 6   Cooking Time: 30 Minutes
Ingredients:
- 2 racks of lamb. Frenched
- 1 tbsp garlic, crushed
- 1 tbsp rosemary
- 1/2 cup olive oil
- Kitchen twine

Directions:
Preheat your   to 450F.   Rinse the lab with clean cold water then pat it dry with a paper towel.   Lay the lamb flat on a chopping board and score a ¼ inch down between the bones. Repeat the process between the bones on each lamb rack. Set aside.   In a small mixing bowl, combine garlic, rosemary, and oil. Brush the lamb of rack generously with the mixture.   Bend the lamb rack into a semicircle then place the racks together such that the bones will be up and will form a crown shape. Wrap around 4 times starting from the base moving upward. Tie tightly to keep the racks together.   Place the lambs on a baking sheet and set in the . Cook on high heat for 10 minutes. Reduce the temperature to 300F and cook for 20 more minutes or until the internal temperature reaches 130F.   Remove the lamb rack from the   and let rest while wrapped in a foil for 15 minutes.   Serve when hot.
Nutrition Info: Calories 390, Total fat 35g, Saturated fat 15g, Total carbs 0g, Net carbs 0g Protein 17g, Sugars 0g, Fiber 0g, Sodium 65mg

340. Wood Pellet Smoked Pork Ribs

Servings: 4   Cooking Time: 10 Hours
Ingredients:
- 2 racks baby back ribs
- 1 cup homemade BBQ rub
- 24 oz hard apple cider
- 1 cup dark brown sugar
- 2 batches homemade BBQ sauce

Directions:
Set your wood pellet to smoke.   Remove the membrane from the pork ribs then generously coat with bbq sauce.   Smoke at 175°F for 5 hours. Increase the grill temperature to 225°F.   Transfer the pork to a high sided pan that has been sprayed with cooking spray. Pour over the apple cider and rub the pork with sugar. Cover the pan with foil and place it back to the grill. Cook for 4 more hours.   Transfer the ribs from the pan to the grill grate and increase the temperature to 300°F.

Brush the ribs with BBQ sauce 3 times in the next 1 hour. Remove the ribs from the grill and serve them. Enjoy.
Nutrition Info: Calories 1073, Total fat 42g, Saturated fat 15g, Total Carbs 111g, Net Carbs 108g, Protein 61g, Sugar 99g, Fiber 3g, Sodium: 1663mg

341. Sweet Smoked Country Ribs

Servings: 12 To 15   Cooking Time: 4 Hours
Ingredients:
- 2 pounds country-style ribs
- 1 batch Sweet Brown Sugar Rub
- 2 tablespoons light brown sugar
- 1 cup Pepsi or other cola
- ¼ cup The Ultimate BBQ Sauce

Directions:
Supply your smoker with wood pellets and follow the manufacturer's specific start-up procedure. Preheat the grill, with the lid closed, to 180°F.   Sprinkle the ribs with the rub and use your hands to work the rub into the meat.   Place the ribs directly on the grill grate and smoke for 3 hours.   Remove the ribs from the grill and place them on enough aluminum foil to wrap them completely. Dust the brown sugar over the ribs. Increase the grill's temperature to 300°F.   Fold in three sides of the foil around the ribs and add the cola. Fold in the last side, completely enclosing the ribs and liquid. Return the ribs to the grill and cook for 45 minutes. Remove the ribs from the foil and place them on the grill grate. Baste all sides of the ribs with barbecue sauce. Cook for 15 minutes more to caramelize the sauce. Remove the ribs from the grill and serve immediately.

342. Boneless Leg Of Lamb

Servings: 4   Cooking Time: 4 Hours
Ingredients:
- 2 1/2 pounds leg of lamb, boneless, fat trimmed
- For the Marinade:
- 2 teaspoons minced garlic
- 1 tablespoon ground black pepper
- 2 tablespoons salt
- 1 teaspoon thyme
- 2 tablespoons oregano
- 2 tablespoons olive oil

Directions:
Take a small bowl, place all the ingredients for the marinade in it and then stir until combined.   Rub the marinade on all sides of lamb, then place it in a large sheet, cover with a plastic wrap and marinate for a minimum of 1 hour in the refrigerator.   When ready to cook, switch on the   grill, fill the grill hopper with apple-flavored wood pellets, power the grill on by using the control panel, select 'smoke' on the temperature dial, or set the temperature to 250 degrees F and let it preheat for a minimum of 5 minutes.   Meanwhile,   When the grill has preheated, open the lid, place the lamb on the grill grate, shut the grill and smoke for 4 hours until the internal temperature reaches 145 degrees F.

When done, transfer lamb to a cutting board, let it stand for 10 minutes, then carve it into slices and serve.
Nutrition Info: Calories: 213 Cal ;Fat: 9 g ;Carbs: 1 g ;Protein: 29 g ;Fiber: 0 g

343. Competition Style Bbq Pork Ribs

Servings: 6   Cooking Time: 2 Hours
Ingredients:
- 2 racks of St. Louis-style ribs
- 1 cup   Pork and Poultry Rub
- 1/8 cup brown sugar
- 4 tablespoons butter
- 4 tablespoons agave
- 1 bottle   Sweet and Heat BBQ Sauce

Directions:
Place the ribs in working surface and remove the thin film of connective tissues covering it. In a smaller bowl, combine the   Pork and Poultry Rub, brown sugar, butter, and agave. Mix until well combined.   Massage the rub onto the ribs and allow to rest in the fridge for at least 2 hours.   When ready to cook, fire the   Grill to 225F. Use desired wood pellets when cooking the ribs. Close the lid and preheat for 15 minutes.   Place the ribs on the grill grate and close the lid. Smoke for 1 hour and 30 minutes. Make sure to flip the ribs halfway through the cooking time.   Ten minutes before the cooking time ends, brush the ribs with BBQ sauce.   Remove from the grill and allow to rest before slicing.
Nutrition Info: Calories per serving: 399 ;
Protein: 47.2g; Carbs: 3.5g; Fat: 20.5g Sugar: 2.3g

344. Smoked And Pulled Beef

Servings: 6   Cooking Time: 6 Hours
Ingredients:
- 4 lb beef sirloin tip roast
- 1/2 cup bbq rub
- 2 bottles of amber beer
- 1 bottle barbecues sauce

Directions:
Turn your wood pellet grill onto smoke setting then trim excess fat from the steak.   Coat the steak with bbq rub and let it smoke on the grill for 1 hour.   Continue cooking and flipping the steak for the next 3 hours. Transfer the steak to a braising vessel .add the beers. Braise the beef until tender then transfer to a platter reserving 2 cups of cooking liquid.   Use a pair of forks to shred the beef and return it to the pan. Add the reserved liquid and barbecue sauce. Stir well and keep warm before serving.   Enjoy.
Nutrition Info: Calories 829, Total fat 46g, Saturated fat 18g, Total carbs 4g, Net carbs 4g, Protein 86g, Sugar 0g, Fiber 0g, Sodium: 181mg

345. Pastrami Short Ribs

Servings: 4   Cooking Time: 3 ½ Hours
Ingredients:

- 2 quarts water
- 1/3 cup salt
- 2 teaspoon pink salt
- ¼ cup brown sugar
- 4 garlic
- 4 tablespoons coriander seeds
- 3 tablespoons peppercorns
- 2 teaspoons mustard seeds
- 2 tablespoons extra virgin olive oil
- 1 large ginger ale
- 2 pounds beef short ribs

Directions:
Place all ingredients except for the oil, ginger ale, and short ribs in a large bowl. Mix until well-combined. Add in the short ribs. Marinate the short ribs in the fridge for at least 12 hours.   When ready to cook, fire the   Grill to 300F. Use desired wood pellets when cooking. Close the lid and preheat for 15 minutes.   Place the short ribs on the grill grate and smoke for 2 hours. Drizzle with oil.   Transfer the ribs on a roasting pan and pour enough ginger ale all over the ribs. Cover the pan with foil.   Place in the grill and increase the temperature to 350F and cook for 1 ½ hours.
Nutrition Info: Calories per serving: 521 ;
Protein: 46.7g; Carbs: 16.9g; Fat: 30.1g Sugar: 13.7g

346. Grilled Pork Tenderloin With Herb Sauce

Servings: 4   Cooking Time: 15 Minutes
Ingredients:
- 1 pork tenderloin
- Bbq seasoning
- Fresh Herb Sauce
- 1 handful basil, fresh
- 1/2 handful flat-leaf parsley, fresh
- 1/4 tbsp garlic powder
- 1/3 cup olive oil
- 1/2 tbsp kosher salt

Directions:
Preheat your   to medium heat.   Remove silver skin from the pork tenderloin and pat it dry with a paper towel.   Generously rub the pork with the bbq seasoning then cook over indirect heat in the   while turning occasionally.   Cook until the internal temperature reaches 145F. Remove the pork from the   and let rest for 10 minutes.   Meanwhile, add all the fresh herb sauce ingredients in a food processor and pulse a few times.   Slice the pork tenderloin diagonally and spoon the sauce on top. Serve
Nutrition Info: Calories 300, Total fat 22g, Saturated fat 4g, Total carbs 13g, Net carbs 12g Protein 14g, Sugars 10g, Fiber 1g, Sodium 791mg

347. Smoked Apple Bbq Ribs

Servings: 6   Cooking Time: 2 Hours
Ingredients:
- 2 racks St. Louis-style ribs
- ¼ cup   Big Game Rub

- 1 cup apple juice
- A bottle of BBQ Sauce

Directions:
Place the ribs on a working surface and remove the film of connective tissues covering it. In another bowl, mix the Game Rub and apple juice until well-combined. Massage the rub on to the ribs and allow to rest in the fridge for at least 2 hours. When ready to cook, fire the Grill to 225F. Use apple wood pellets when cooking the ribs. Close the lid and preheat for 15 minutes. Place the ribs on the grill grate and close the lid. Smoke for 1 hour and 30 minutes. Make sure to flip the ribs halfway through the cooking time. Ten minutes before the cooking time ends, brush the ribs with BBQ sauce. Remove from the grill and allow to rest before slicing.

Nutrition Info: Calories per serving: 337 ;
Protein: 47.1g; Carbs: 4.7 g; Fat: 12.9g Sugar: 4g

348. Traditional Tomahawk Steak

Servings: 4 To 6   Cooking Time: 1 Or 2 Hours
Ingredients:
- 1 tomahawk ribeye steak (2 1/2 to 3 1/2 lbs)
- 5 garlic cloves, minced
- 2 tbsp kosher salt
- 1 bundle fresh thyme
- 2 tbsp ground black pepper
- 8 oz butter stick
- 1 tbsp garlic powder
- 1/8 cup olive oil

Directions:
Mix rub ingredients (salt, black pepper, and garlic powder) in a small bowl. Use this mixture to season all sides of the ribeye steak generously. You can also substitute your favorite steak seasoning. After applying seasoning, let the steak rest at room temperature for at least 30 minutes. While the steak rests, preheat your pellet grill to 450°F - 550°F for searing   Sear the steak for 5 minutes on each side. Halfway through each side (so after 2 1/2 minutes), rotate the steak 90° to form grill marks on the tomahawk   After the tomahawk steak has seared for 5 minutes on each side (10 minutes total), move the steak to a raised rack   Adjust your pellet grill's temperature to 250°F and turn up smoke setting if applicable. Leave the lid open for a moment to help allow some heat to escape   Stick your probe meat thermometer into the very center of the cut to measure internal temperature.   Place butter stick, garlic cloves, olive oil, and thyme in the aluminum pan. Then place the aluminum pan under the steak to catch drippings. After a few minutes, the steak drippings and ingredients will mix together   Baste the steak with the aluminum pan mixture every 10 minutes until the tomahawk steak reaches your desired doneness   Once the steak reaches its desired doneness, remove from the grill and place on a cutting board or serving dish. The steak should rest for 10-15 minutes before cutting/serving.

349. Teriyaki Pork Tenderloin

Servings: 12 To 15   Cooking Time: 1½ To 2 Hours
Ingredients:
- 2 (1-pound) pork tenderloins
- 1 batch Quick and Easy Teriyaki Marinade
- Smoked salt

Directions:
In a large zip-top bag, combine the tenderloins and marinade. Seal the bag, turn to coat, and refrigerate the pork for at least 30 minutes—I recommend up to overnight.   Supply your smoker with wood pellets and follow the manufacturer's specific start-up procedure. Preheat the grill, with the lid closed, to 180°F.   Remove the tenderloins from the marinade and season them with smoked salt.   Place the tenderloins directly on the grill grate and smoke for 1 hour.   Increase the grill's temperature to 300°F and continue to cook until the pork's internal temperature reaches 145°F.   Remove the tenderloins from the grill and let them rest for 5 to 10 minutes, before thinly slicing and serving.

350. Tri-tip

Servings: 6   Cooking Time: 1 Hour 30 Minutes;
Ingredients:
- 3 lb tri-tip
- 1-1/2 tbsp kosher salt
- 1 tbsp black pepper
- 1 tbsp paprika
- 1/2 tbsp cayenne
- 1 tbsp onion powder
- 1 tbsp garlic powder

Directions:
Preheat your   to 250F.   Mix the seasoning ingredients and generously season the tri-tip.   Place it in the   and cook for 30 minutes. Flip the tri-tip and cook for an additional 30 minutes.   Turn up the   and coo for additional 30 minutes. Pull out the meat at 125F for medium-rare and 135F for medium.   Let the meat rest for 10 minutes before slicing and serving.

Nutrition Info: Calories 484, Total fat 25g, Saturated fat 0g, Total carbs 1g, Net carbs 1g Protein 59g, Sugars 0g, Fiber 0g, Sodium 650mmg

351. Smoked Pulled Lamb Sliders

Servings: 7   Cooking Time: 9 Hours
Ingredients:
- 5 lb. lamb shoulder, boneless
- 1/2 cup olive oil
- 1/3 cup kosher salt
- 1/3 cup pepper, coarsely ground
- 1/3 cup granulated garlic
- For the spritz
- 4 oz Worcestershire sauce
- 6 oz apple cider vinegar

Directions:
Preheat the   to 225F with a pan of water for moisture. Trim any excess fat from the lamb then pat it dry with

some paper towel. Rub with oil, salt, pepper, and garlic. Place the lamb in the smoker for 90 minutes then spritz every 30 minutes until the internal temperature reaches 165F. Transfer the lamb in a foil pan then add the remaining spritz liquid. Cover with a foil and place back in the . Smoke until the internal temperature reaches 205F. Remove from the smoker and let rest in a cooler without ice for 30 minutes before pulling it. Serve with slaw or bun and enjoy.

Nutrition Info: Calories 235, Total fat 6g, Saturated fat 1g, Total carbs 22g, Net carbs 21g Protein 20g, Sugars 7g, Fiber 1g, Sodium 592mg, Potassium 318mg

352. 2-ingredients Filet Mignon

Servings: 2   Cooking Time: 10 Minutes
Ingredients:
- 2 filet mignons
- Salt and freshly ground black pepper, to taste

Directions:
Set the temperature of Grill to 450 degrees F and preheat with closed lid for 15 minutes. Season the steaks with salt and black pepper generously. Place the filet mignons onto the grill and grill and cook for about 5 minutes per side. Remove from grill and serve immediately.

Nutrition Info: Calories per serving: 254; Carbohydrates: 0g; Protein: 39.8g; Fat: 9.3g; Sugar: 0g; Sodium: 161mg; Fiber: 0g

353. Grilled Venison Kabob

Servings: 6   Cooking Time: 15 Minutes
Ingredients:
- 1 venison, black strap steaks cut into large cubes
- 2 whole red onion, quartered
- 2 whole green bell pepper, sliced into big squares
- Oil as needs
- Salt and pepper to taste

Directions:
Place all ingredients in a mixing bowl. Toss to coat the meat and vegetables with the oil and seasoning. Thread the meat and vegetables into metal skewers in an alternating manner. Fire the Grill to 500F. Use desired wood pellets when cooking. Close the lid and preheat for 15 minutes. Place the kabobs on the grill grate and cook for 15 minutes. Make sure to turn once halfway through the cooking time. Remove from the grill and serve with yogurt if desired.

Nutrition Info: Calories per serving: 267; Protein: 32.4g; Carbs: 10.1g; Fat: 10.4g Sugar:4.8 g

354. Thai Beef Salad

Servings: 4   Cooking Time: 10 Minutes
Ingredients:
- 1 ½ pound skirt steak
- 1 ½ teaspoon salt
- 1 teaspoon ground white pepper

- For the Dressing:
- 4 jalapeño peppers, minced
- ½ teaspoon minced garlic
- 4 tablespoons Thai fish sauce
- 4 tablespoons lime juice
- 1 tablespoon brown sugar
- For the Salad:
- 1 small red onion, peeled, thinly sliced
- 6 cherry tomatoes, halved
- 2 green onions, ¼-inch diced
- 1 cucumber, deseeded, thinly sliced
- 1 heart of romaine lettuce, chopped
- ½ cup chopped mint
- 2 tablespoons cilantro
- ½ teaspoon red pepper flakes
- 1 tablespoon lime juice
- 2 tablespoons fish sauce

Directions:
Switch on the grill, fill the grill hopper with cherry flavored wood pellets, power the grill on by using the control panel, select 'smoke' on the temperature dial, or set the temperature to 450 degrees F and let it preheat for a minimum of 15 minutes. Meanwhile, prepare the steak, and for this, season it with salt and black pepper until well coated. When the grill has preheated, open the lid, place steak on the grill grate, shut the grill and smoke for 10 minutes until internal temperature reaches 130 degrees F. Meanwhile, prepare the dressing and for this, take a medium bowl, place all of its ingredients in it and then stir until combined. Take a large salad, place all the ingredients for the salad in it, drizzle with dressing and toss until well coated and mixed. When done, transfer steak to a cutting board, let it rest for 10 minutes and then cut it into slices. Add steak slices into the salad, toss until mixed, and then serve.

Nutrition Info: Calories: 128 Cal ;Fat: 6 g ;Carbs: 6 g ;Protein: 12 g ;Fiber: 1 g

355. Grilled Lamb Kabobs

Servings: 7   Cooking Time: 16 Minutes
Ingredients:
- ½ cup olive oil
- ½ tablespoon salt
- 2 teaspoons black pepper
- 2 tablespoons chopped mint
- ½ tablespoon cilantro, chopped
- 1 teaspoon cumin
- ½ cup lemon juice
- 3 pounds boneless leg of lamb, cut into 2-inch cubes
- 15 apricots, halved and seeded
- 5 onions, cut into wedges

Directions:
In a bowl, combine the oil, salt, pepper, mint, cilantro, cumin, and lemon juice. Massage the mixture on to the lamb shoulder and allow to marinate in the fridge for at least 2 hours. Remove the lamb from the marinade and thread the lamb, apricots, and red onion alternatingly on a skewer. When ready to cook, fire the Grill to 400F. Use desired wood pellets when

cooking. Close the lid and preheat for 15 minutes. Place the skewers on the grill grate and cook for 8 minutes on each side. Remove from the grill.

Nutrition Info: Calories per serving: 652; Protein: 53.9g; Carbs: 38.1g; Fat: 31.8g Sugar: 29.4g

356. Braised Pork Chile Verde

Servings: 6 Cooking Time: 40 Minutes

Ingredients:
- 3 pounds pork shoulder, bone removed and cut into ½ inch cubes
- 1 tablespoon all-purpose flour
- Salt and pepper to taste
- 1-pound tomatillos, husked and washed
- 2 jalapenos, chopped
- 1 medium yellow onion, peeled and cut into chunks
- 4 cloves of garlic
- 4 tablespoons extra virgin olive oil
- 2 cup chicken stock
- 2 cans green chilies
- 1 tablespoon cumin
- 1 tablespoon oregano
- ½ lime, juiced
- ¼ cup cilantro

Directions:
Place the pork shoulder chunks in a bowl and toss with flour. Season with salt and pepper to taste. When ready to cook, fire the Grill to 500F. Use desired wood pellets when cooking. Place a large cast iron skillet on the bottom rack of the grill. Close the lid and preheat for 15 minutes. Place the tomatillos, jalapeno, onion, and garlic on a sheet tray lined with foil and drizzle with 2 tablespoon olive oil. Season with salt and pepper to taste. Place the remaining olive oil in the heated cast iron skillet and cook the pork shoulder. Spread the meat evenly then close. Before closing the lid, place the vegetables in the tray on the grill rack. Close the lid of the grill. Cook for 20 minutes without opening the lid or stirring the pork. After 20 minutes, remove the vegetables from the grill and transfer to a blender. Pulse until smooth and pour into the pan with the pork. Stir in the chicken stock, green chilies, cumin, oregano, and lime juice. Season with salt and pepper to taste. Close the grill lid and cook for another 20 minutes. Once cooked, stir in the cilantro.

Nutrition Info: Calories per serving: 389; Protein: 28.5g; Carbs: 4.5g; Fat: 24.3g Sugar: 2.1g

357. Bbq Baby Back Ribs

Servings: 8 Cooking Time: 6 Hours

Ingredients:
- 2 racks of baby back pork ribs, membrane removed
- Pork and poultry rub as needed
- 1/2 cup brown sugar
- 1/3 cup honey, warmed
- 1/3 cup yellow mustard

- 1 tablespoon Worcestershire sauce
- 1 cup BBQ sauce
- 1/2 cup apple juice, divided

Directions:
Switch on the grill, fill the grill hopper with hickory flavored wood pellets, power the grill on by using the control panel, select 'smoke' on the temperature dial, or set the temperature to 180 degrees F and let it preheat for a minimum of 15 minutes. Meanwhile, take a small bowl, place mustard, and Worcestershire sauce in it, pour in ¼ cup apple juice and whisk until combined and smooth paste comes together. Brush this paste on all sides of ribs and then season with pork and poultry rub until coated. When the grill has preheated, open the lid, place ribs on the grill grate meat-side up, shut the grill and smoke for 3 hours. After 3 hours, transfer ribs to a rimmed baking dish, let rest for 15 minutes, and meanwhile, change the smoking temperature of the grill to 225 degrees F and let it preheat for a minimum of 10 minutes. Then return pork into the rimmed baking sheet to the grill grate and cook for 3 minutes per side until slightly charred. When done, remove the baking sheet from the grill and work on one rib at a time, sprinkle half of the sugar over the rib, drizzle with half of the honey and half of the remaining apple juice, cover with aluminum foil to seal completely. Repeat with the remaining ribs, return foiled ribs on the grill grate, shut with lid, and then smoke for 2 hours. After 2 hours, uncover the grill, brush them with BBQ sauce generously, arrange them on the grill grate and grill for 1 hour until glazed. When done, transfer ribs to a cutting board, let it rest for 15 minutes, slice into pieces and then serve.

Nutrition Info: Calories: 334 Cal ;Fat: 22.5 g ;Carbs: 6.5 g ;Protein: 24 g ;Fiber: 0.1 g

358. Smoked Ham

Servings: 12 To 15 Cooking Time: 5 Or 6 Hours

Ingredients:
- 1 (10-pound) fresh ham, skin removed
- 2 tablespoons olive oil
- 1 batch Rosemary-Garlic Lamb Seasoning

Directions:
Supply your smoker with wood pellets and follow the manufacturer's specific start-up procedure. Preheat the grill, with the lid closed, to 180°F. Rub the ham all over with olive oil and sprinkle it with the seasoning. Place the ham directly on the grill grate and smoke for 3 hours. Increase the grill's temperature to 375°F and continue to smoke the ham until its internal temperature reaches 170°F. Remove the ham from the grill and let it rest for 10 minutes, before carving and serving.

359. Roasted Pork With Blackberry Sauce

Servings: 4 Cooking Time: 50 Minutes

Ingredients:
- 2 lb. pork tenderloin
- 2 tablespoons dried rosemary

- Salt and pepper to taste
- 2 tablespoons olive oil
- 12 blackberries, sliced
- 1 cup balsamic vinegar
- 4 tablespoons sugar

Directions:
Preheat the wood pellet grill to 350 degrees F for 15 minutes while the lid is closed. Season the pork with the rosemary, salt and pepper. In a pan over high heat, pour in the oil and sear pork for 2 minutes per side. Transfer to the grill and cook for 20 minutes. Take the pan off the grill. Let rest for 10 minutes. In a pan over medium heat, simmer the blackberries in vinegar and sugar for 30 minutes. Pour sauce over the pork and serve. Tips: You can also simmer the pork in the blackberry sauce for 10 minutes.

360. Smoked Lamb Meatballs

Servings: 20   Cooking Time: 1 Hour
Ingredients:
- 1 lb. lamb shoulder, ground
- 3 garlic cloves, finely diced
- 3 tbsp. shallot, diced
- 1 tbsp. salt
- 1 egg
- 1/2 tbsp. pepper
- 1/2 tbsp. cumin
- 1/2 tbsp. smoked paprika
- 1/4 tbsp. red pepper flakes
- 1/4 tbsp. cinnamon
- 1/4 cup panko breadcrumbs

Directions:
Set your to 250F . Combine all the ingredients in a small bowl then mix thoroughly using your hands. Form golf ball-sized meatballs and place them in a baking sheet. Place the baking sheet in the smoker and smoke until the internal temperature reaches 160F. Remove the meatballs from the smoker and serve when hot.
Nutrition Info: Calories 93, Total fat 5.9g, Saturated fat 2.5g, Total carbs 4.8g, Net carbs 4.5g Protein 5g, Sugars 0.3g, Fiber 0.3g, Sodium 174.1mg, Potassium 82.8mg

361. Leg Of A Lamb

Servings: 10   Cooking Time: 2 Hours And 30 Minutes
Ingredients:
- 1 (8-ounce) package softened cream cheese
- ¼ cup cooked and crumbled bacon
- 1 seeded and chopped jalapeño pepper
- 1 tablespoon crushed dried rosemary
- 2 teaspoons garlic powder
- 1 teaspoon onion powder
- 1 teaspoon paprika
- 1 teaspoon cayenne pepper
- Salt, to taste
- 1 (4-5-pound) butterflied leg of lamb
- 2-3 tablespoons olive oil

Directions:
For filling in a bowl, add all ingredients and mix till well combined. For spice mixture in another small bowl, mix together all ingredients. Place the leg of lamb onto a smooth surface. Sprinkle the inside of leg with some spice mixture. Place filling mixture over the inside surface evenly. Roll the leg of lamb tightly and with a butcher's twine, tie the roll to secure the filling Coat the outer side of roll with olive oil evenly and then sprinkle with spice mixture. Preheat the pallet grill to 225-240 degrees F. Arrange the leg of lamb in pallet grill and cook for about 2-2½ hours. Remove the leg of lamb from pallet grill and transfer onto a cutting board. With a piece of foil, cover leg loosely and transfer onto a cutting board for about 20-25 minutes before slicing. With a sharp knife, cut the leg of lamb in desired sized slices and serve.
Nutrition Info: Calories: 715 Cal Fat: 38.9 g Carbohydrates: 2.2 g   Protein: 84.6 g Fiber: 0.1 g

362. Wood Pellet Grilled Pork Chops

Servings: 6   Cooking Time: 10 Minutes
Ingredients:
- 6 pork chops, thickly cut
- BBQ rub

Directions:
Preheat the wood pellet to 450°F. Season the pork chops generously with the bbq rub. Place the pork chops on the grill and cook for 6 minutes or until the internal temperature reaches 145°F. Remove from the grill and let sit for 10 minutes before serving. Enjoy.
Nutrition Info: Calories 264, Total fat 13g, Saturated fat 6g, Total Carbs 4g, Net Carbs 1g, Protein 33g, Sugar 0g, Fiber 3g, Sodium: 66mg

363. Braised Mediterranean Beef Brisket

Servings: 16   Cooking Time: 5 Hours
Ingredients:
- 3 tablespoons dried rosemary
- 2 tablespoons cumin seeds, ground
- 2 tablespoons dried coriander
- 1 tablespoon dried oregano
- 2 teaspoons ground cinnamon
- ½ teaspoon salt
- 8 pounds beef brisket, sliced into chunks
- 1 cup beef stock

Directions:
Mix the rosemary, cumin, coriander, oregano, cinnamon, and salt in a bowl. Massage the spice mix into the beef brisket and allow to rest in the fridge for 12 hours. When ready to cook, fire the Grill to 180F. Use desired wood pellets when cooking. Close the lid and preheat for 15 minutes. Place the brisket fat side down on the grill grate and cook for 4 hours. After 4 hours, turn up the heat to 250F. Continue cooking the beef brisket until the internal temperature reaches 160F. Remove and place on a foil. Crimp the edges of the foil to create a sleeve. Pour in the beef stock. Return the

brisket in the foil sleeve and continue cooking for another hour.

Nutrition Info: Calories per serving: 453 ;
Protein: 33.5g; Carbs: 1g; Fat: 34g Sugar: 0.1g

364. Grilled Leg Of Lamb Steak

Servings: 4   Cooking Time: 10 Minutes
Ingredients:
- 4 eaches lamb steaks, bone-in
- 1/4 cup olive oil
- 4 garlic cloves, minced
- 1 tbsp rosemary, freshly chopped
- Salt and pepper to taste

Directions:
Arrange the steak in a dish in a single layer. Cover the meat with oil, garlic, fresh rosemary, salt, and pepper. Flip the meat to coat on all sides and let it marinate. For 30 minutes.   Preheat your   and lightly oil the grates cook the meat on the grill until well browned on both sides and the internal temperature reaches 140F. Serve and enjoy.

Nutrition Info: Calories 327.3, Total fat 21.9g, Saturated fat 5.3g, Total carbs 1.7g, Net carbs 1.5g Protein 29.6g, Sugars 0.1g, Fiber 0.2g, Sodium 112.1mg, Potassium 409.8mg

365. Baby Back Ribs

Servings: 12 To 15   Cooking Time: 5 To 6 Hours
Ingredients:
- 2 full slabs baby back ribs, back membranes removed
- 1 cup prepared table mustard
- 1 cup Pork Rub
- 1 cup apple juice, divided
- 1 cup packed light brown sugar, divided
- 1 cup of The Ultimate BBQ Sauce, divided

Directions:
Supply your   with wood pellets and follow the manufacturer's specific start-up procedure. Preheat, with the lid closed, to 150° to 180°F, or to the "Smoke" setting.   Coat the ribs with the mustard to help the rub stick and lock in moisture.   Generously apply the rub Place the ribs directly on the grill, close the lid, and smoke for 3 hoursIncrease the temperature to 225°F. Remove the ribs from the grill and wrap each rack individually with aluminum foil, but before sealing tightly, add ½ cup apple juice and ½ cup brown sugar to each package   Return the foil-wrapped ribs to the grill, close the lid, and smoke for 2 more hours.   Carefully unwrap the ribs and remove the foil completely. Coat each slab with ½ cup of barbecue sauce and continue smoking with the lid closed for 30 minutes to 1 hour, or until the meat tightens and has a reddish bark. For the perfect rack, the internal temperature should be 190°F.

366. Spicy & Tangy Lamb Shoulder

Servings: 6   Cooking Time: 5¾ Hours
Ingredients:
- 1 (5-lb.) bone-in lamb shoulder, trimmed
- 3-4 tbsp. Moroccan seasoning
- 2 tbsp. olive oil
- 1 C. water
- ¼ C. apple cider vinegar

Directions:
Set the temperature of   Grill to 275 degrees F and preheat with closed lid for 15 minutes, using charcoal. Coat the lamb shoulder with oil evenly and then rub with Moroccan seasoning generously.   Place the lamb shoulder onto the grill and cook for about 45 minutes. In a food-safe spray bottle, mix together vinegar and water.   Spray the lamb shoulder with vinegar mixture evenly.   Cook for about 4-5 hours, spraying with vinegar mixture after every 20 minutes.   Remove the lamb shoulder from grill and place onto a cutting board for about 20 minutes before slicing.   With a sharp knife, cut the lamb shoulder in desired sized slices and serve.

Nutrition Info: Calories per serving: 563;
Carbohydrates: 3.1g; Protein: 77.4g; Fat: 25.2g; Sugar: 1.4g; Sodium: 1192mg; Fiber: 0g

367. Wood Pellet Togarashi Pork Tenderloin

Servings: 6   Cooking Time: 25 Minutes
Ingredients:
- 1 Pork tenderloin
- 1/2tbsp kosher salt
- 1/4 cup Togarashi seasoning

Directions:
Cut any excess silver skin from the pork and sprinkle with salt to taste. Rub generously with the togarashi seasoning   Place in a preheated oven at 400°F for 25 minutes or until the internal temperature reaches 145°F. Remove from the grill and let rest for 10 minutes before slicing and serving.   Enjoy.

Nutrition Info: Calories 390, Total fat 13g, Saturated fat 6g, Total Carbs 4g, Net Carbs 1g, Protein 33g, Sugar 0g, Fiber 3g, Sodium: 66mg

368. Cheesy Lamb Burgers

Servings: 4   Cooking Time: 20 Minutes
Ingredients:
- 2 lb. ground lamb
- 1 C. Parmigiano-Reggiano cheese, grated
- Salt and freshly ground black pepper, to taste

Directions:
Set the temperature of   Grill to 425 degrees F and preheat with closed lid for 15 minutes.   In a bowl, add all ingredients and mix well.   Make 4 (¾-inch thick) patties from mixture.   With your thumbs, make a shallow but wide depression in each patty.   Arrange the patties onto the grill, depression-side down and cook

for about 8 minutes.   Flip and cook for about 8-10 minutes.   Serve immediately.
Nutrition Info: Calories per serving: 502; Carbohydrates: 0g; Protein: 71.7g; Fat: 22.6g; Sugar: 0g; Sodium: 331mg; Fiber: 0g

369. Simple Wood Pellet Smoked Pork Ribs

Servings: 7   Cooking Time: 5 Hours
Ingredients:
- 3 rack baby back ribs
- 3/4 cup pork and poultry rub
- 3/4 cup Que BBQ Sauce

Directions:
Peel the membrane from the backside of the ribs and trim any fat.   Season the pork generously with the rub. Set the wood pellet grill to 180°F and preheat for 15 minutes with the lid closed.   Place the pork ribs on the grill and smoke them for 5 hours.   Remove the pork from the grill and wrap them in a foil with the BBQ sauce. Place back the pork and increase the temperature to 350°F. Cook for 45 more minutes.   Remove the pork from the grill and let it rest for 20 minutes before serving. Enjoy.
Nutrition Info: Calories 762, Total fat 57g, Saturated fat 17g, Total Carbs 23g, Net Carbs 22.7g, Protein 39g, Sugar 18g, Fiber 0.5g, Sodium: 737mg, Potassium 618mg

370. Pickled-pepper Pork Chops

Servings: 4   Cooking Time: 45 To 50 Minutes
Ingredients:
- 4 (1-inch-thick) pork chops
- ½ cup pickled jalapeño juice or pickle juice
- ¼ cup chopped pickled (jarred) jalapeño pepper slices
- ¼ cup chopped roasted red peppers
- ¼ cup canned diced tomatoes, well-drained
- ¼ cup chopped scallions
- 2 teaspoons poultry seasoning
- 2 teaspoons salt
- 2 teaspoons freshly ground black pepper

Directions:
Pour the jalapeño juice into a large container with a lid. Add the pork chops, cover, and marinate in the refrigerator for at least 4 hours or overnight, supplementing with or substituting pickle juice as desired.   In a small bowl, combine the chopped pickled jalapeños, roasted red peppers, tomatoes, scallions, and poultry seasoning to make a relish. Set aside.   Remove the pork chops from the marinade and shake off any excess. Discard the marinade. Season both sides of the chops with the salt and pepper.   Supply your smoker with wood pellets and follow the manufacturer's specific start-up procedure. Preheat, with the lid closed, to 325°F.   To serve, divide the chops among plates and top with the pickled pepper relish.

371. Wood Pellet Smoked Brisket

Servings: 10   Cooking Time: 9 Hours
Ingredients:
- 2 tbsp garlic powder
- 2 tbsp onion powder
- 2 tbsp paprika
- 2 tbsp chili powder
- 1/3 cup salt
- 1/3 cup black pepper
- 12 lb whole packer brisket, trimmed
- 1-1/2 cup beef broth

Directions:
Set your wood pellet temperature to 225°F. Let preheat for 15 minutes with the lid closed.   Meanwhile, mix garlic, onion, paprika, chili, salt, and pepper in a mixing bowl.   Season the brisket generously on all sides. Place the meat on the grill with the fat side down and let it cool until the internal temperature reaches 160°F. Remove the meat from the grill and double wrap it with foil. Return it to the grill and cook until the internal temperature reaches 204°F.   Remove from grill, unwrap the brisket and let est for 15 minutes.   Slice and serve.
Nutrition Info: Calories 270, Total fat 20g, Saturated fat 8g, Total Carbs 3g, Net Carbs 3g, Protein 20g, Sugar 1g, Fiber 0g, Sodium: 1220mg

372. Wood Pellet Grill Dale's Lamb

Servings: 8   Cooking Time: 50 Minutes
Ingredients:
- 2/3 cup lemon juice
- 1/2 cup brown sugar
- 1/4 cup Dijon mustard
- 1/4 cup soy sauce
- 1/4 cup olive oil
- 2 garlic cloves, minced
- 1 piece ginger root, freshly sliced
- 1 tbsp salt
- 1/2 tbsp black pepper, ground
- 5 lb leg of lamb, butterflied

Directions:
In a mixing bowl, mix lemon juice, sugar, dijon mustard, sauce, oil, garlic cloves, ginger root, salt, and pepper. Place the lamb in a dish and pour the seasoning mixture over it. Cover the dish and put in a fridge to marinate for 8 hours.   Preheat a wood pellet grill to medium heat. Drain the marinade from the dish and bring it to boil in a small saucepan.   Reduce heat and let simmer while whisking occasionally.   Oil the grill grate and place the lamb on it. Cook for 50 minutes or until the internal temperature reaches 145 F while turning occasionally.   Slice the lamb and cover with the marinade. Serve and enjoy.
Nutrition Info: Calories 451, Total fat 27.2g, Saturated fat 9.5g, Total Carbs 17.8g, Net Carbs 17.6g, Protein 32.4g, Sugar 14g, Fiber 0.2g, Sodium: 1015mg, Potassium 455mg.

373. Bloody Mary Flank Steak

Servings: 3   Cooking Time: 14 Minutes
Ingredients:
- 2 cups   Smoked Bloody Mary Mix or V8 Juice
- ½ cup vodka
- 1 whole lemon, juiced
- 3 cloves garlic, minced
- 1 tablespoon Worcestershire sauce
- 1 teaspoon ground black pepper
- 1 teaspoon celery salt
- ½ cup vegetable oil
- 1 ½ pound flank steak

Directions:
Place all ingredients except for the flank steak in a bowl. Mix until well-combined.   Put the flank steak in a plastic bag and pour half of the marinade over. Marinate for at least 24 hours in the fridge.   When ready to cook, fire the   Grill to 500F. Use desired wood pellets when cooking. Close the lid and preheat for 15 minutes.   Drain the flank steak and pat dry using a paper towel.   Place on the grill grate and cook for 7 minutes on each side.   Meanwhile, place the remaining marinade (unused) in a saucepan and heat until the sauce thickens.   Once the steak is cooked, remove from the grill, and allow to rest for 5 minutes before slicing.   Pour over the sauce.

Nutrition Info: Calories per serving: 719 ;
Protein: 51.9g; Carbs: 15.4g; Fat: 51g Sugar: 6.9g

374. New York Strip

Servings: 6   Cooking Time: 15 Minutes
Ingredients:
- 3 New York strips
- Salt and pepper

Directions:
If the steak is in the fridge, remove it 30 minutes prior to cooking.   Preheat the   to 450F.   Meanwhile, season the steak generously with salt and pepper. Place it on the grill and let it cook for 5 minutes per side or until the internal temperature reaches 1280F.   Rest for 10 minutes.

Nutrition Info: Calories: 198 Cal Fat: 14 g
Carbohydrates: 0 g   Protein: 17 g Fiber: 0 g

375. Smoked Leg

Servings: 6   Cooking Time: 3 Hours
Ingredients:
- 1 leg of lamb, boneless
- 2 tbsp oil
- 4 garlic cloves, minced
- 2 tbsp oregano
- 1 tbsp thyme
- 2 tbsp salt
- 1 tbsp black pepper, freshly ground

Directions:
Trim excess fat from the lamb ensuring you keep the meat in an even thickness for even cooking.   In a mixing bowl, mix oil, garlic, and all spices. Rub the mixture all over the lamb then cover with a plastic wrap. Place the lamb in a fridge and let marinate for an hour. Transfer the lamb on a smoker rack and set the   to smoke at 250F.   Smoke the meat for 4 hours or until the internal temperature reaches 145F   Remove from the   and serve immediately.

Nutrition Info: Calories 356, Total fat 16g, Saturated fat 5g, Total carbs 3g, Net carbs 2g Protein 49g, Sugars 1g, Fiber 1g, Sodium 2474mg

376. Tri-tip Roast

Servings: 6   Cooking Time: 3 Hours And 45 Minutes
Ingredients:
- 1 tri-tip roast
- 'Que BBQ Sauce, as needed
- Prime Rib Rub, as needed
- ½ cup beef broth

Directions:
Marinate the tri-trip roast in the   Que BBQ Sauce overnight inside the fridge.   Once ready to cook, remove the beef from the marinade and season with the Prime Rib Rub.   Fire the   Grill to 180F. Use desired wood pellets when cooking. Close the lid and preheat for 15 minutes.   Place the beef on the grill grate and cook for 3 hours.   Remove from the grill and place the beef on an aluminum foil sheet. Crimp the edges of the aluminum foil to create a sleeve.   Place the roast in the aluminum sleeve on the grill grate and pour over the beef broth.   Pour over the broth and increase the heat to 300F. Cook for 45 minutes.

Nutrition Info: Calories per serving: 357;
Protein: 48g; Carbs: 1.7g; Fat: 16g Sugar: 0g

377. Bacon

Servings: 6   Cooking Time: 25 Minutes
Ingredients:
- 1lb bacon

Directions:
Preheat your   to 375F.   Line a baking sheet with parchment paper then arrange the thick-cut bacon on it in a single layer.   Bake the bacon in the   for 20 minutes. Flip the bacon pieces and cook for 20 more minutes or until the bacon is no longer floppy.   Serve and enjoy.

Nutrition Info: Calories 315, Total fat 10g, Saturated fat 0g, Total carbs 0g, Net carbs 0g Protein 9g, Sugars 0g, Fiber 0g, Sodium 500mg

378. Bacon-swiss Cheesesteak Meatloaf

Servings: 4   Cooking Time: 2 Hours
Ingredients:
- 1 tablespoon canola oil
- 2 garlic cloves, finely chopped
- 1 medium onion, finely chopped

- 1 poblano chile, stemmed, seeded, and finely chopped
- 2 pounds extra-lean ground beef
- 2 tablespoons Montreal steak seasoning
- 1 tablespoon A.Steak Sauce
- ½ pound bacon, cooked and crumbled
- 2 cups shredded Swiss cheese
- 1 egg, beaten
- 2 cups breadcrumbs
- ½ cup Tiger Sauce

Directions:
On your stove top, heat the canola oil in a medium sauté pan over medium-high heat. Add the garlic, onion, and poblano, and sauté for 3 to 5 minutes, or until the onion is just barely translucent   Supply your smoker with wood pellets and follow the manufacturer's specific start-up procedure. Preheat, with the lid closed, to 225°F. In a large bowl, combine the sautéed vegetables, ground beef, steak seasoning, steak sauce, bacon, Swiss cheese, egg, and breadcrumbs. Mix with your hands until well incorporated, then shape into a loaf.   Put the meatloaf in a cast iron skillet and place it on the grill. Close the lid and smoke for 2 hours, or until a meat thermometer inserted in the loaf reads 165°F.   Top with the meatloaf with the Tiger Sauce, remove from the grill, and let rest for about 10 minutes before serving.

379. Pork Belly

Servings: 8   Cooking Time: 3 Hours And 30 Minutes
Ingredients:
- 3 pounds pork belly, skin removed
- Pork and poultry rub as needed
- 4 tablespoons salt
- 1/2 teaspoon ground black pepper

Directions:
Switch on the   grill, fill the grill hopper with apple-flavored wood pellets, power the grill on by using the control panel, select 'smoke' on the temperature dial, or set the temperature to 275 degrees F and let it preheat for a minimum of 15 minutes.   Meanwhile, prepare the pork belly and for this, sprinkle pork and poultry rub, salt, and black pepper on all sides of pork belly until well coated.   When the grill has preheated, open the lid, place the pork belly on the grill grate, shut the grill and smoke for 3 hours and 30 minutes until the internal temperature reaches 200 degrees F.   When done, transfer pork belly to a cutting board, let it rest for 15 minutes, then cut it into slices and serve.
Nutrition Info: Calories: 430 Cal ;Fat: 44 g ;Carbs: 1 g ;Protein: 8 g ;Fiber: 0 g

380. Lamb Skewers

Servings: 6   Cooking Time: 8-12 Minutes
Ingredients:
- One lemon, juiced
- Two crushed garlic cloves
- Two chopped red onions
- One t. chopped thyme

- Pepper
- Salt
- One t. oregano
- 1/3 c. oil
- ½ t. cumin
- Two pounds cubed lamb leg

Directions:
Refrigerate the chunked lamb.   The remaining ingredients should be mixed together. Add in the meat. Refrigerate overnight.   Pat the meat dry and thread onto some metal or wooden skewers. Wooden skewers should be soaked in water.   Add wood pellets to your smoker and follow your cooker's startup procedure. Preheat your smoker, with your lid closed, until it reaches 450.   Grill, covered, for 4-6 minutes on each side.   Serve.
Nutrition Info: Calories: 201 Cal Fat: 9 g Carbohydrates: 3 g   Protein: 24 g Fiber: 1 g

381. Holiday Dinner Leg Of Lamb

Servings: 8   Cooking Time: 5 Hours
Ingredients:
- ½ C. olive oil
- ½ C. red wine vinegar
- ½ C. dry white wine
- 1 tbsp. garlic, minced
- 1 tsp. dried marjoram, crushed
- 1 tsp. dried rosemary, crushed
- Salt and freshly ground black pepper, to taste
- 1 (5-lb.) leg of lamb

Directions:
In a bowl, add all ingredients except for leg of lamb and mix until well combined.   In a large resealable bag, add marinade and leg of lamb.   Seal the bag and shake to coat completely.   Refrigerate for about 4-6 hours, flipping occasionally.   Set the temperature of Grill to 225 degrees F and preheat with closed lid for 15 minutes. Place the leg of lamb onto the grill and cook for about 4-5 hours.   Remove the leg of lamb from grill and place onto a cutting board for about 20 minutes before slicing. With a sharp knife, cut the leg of lamb into desired-sized slices and serve.
Nutrition Info: Calories per serving: 653; Carbohydrates: 1g; Protein: 79.7g; Fat: 33.4g; Sugar: 0.2g; Sodium: 237mg; Fiber: 0.1g

382. Korean Style Bbq Prime Ribs

Servings: 5   Cooking Time: 8 Hours
Ingredients:
- 3 lbs beef short ribs
- 2 tbsp sugar
- 3/4 cup water
- 1 tbsp ground black pepper
- 3 tbsp white vinegar
- 2 tbsp sesame oil
- 3 tbsp soy sauce
- 6 cloves garlic, minced
- 1/3 cup light brown sugar

- 1/2 yellow onion, finely chopped

Directions:
Combine soy sauce, water, and vinegar in a bowl. Mix and whisk in brown sugar, white sugar, pepper, sesame oil, garlic, and onion. Whisk until the sugars have completely dissolved   Pour marinade into large bowl or baking pan with high sides. Dunk the short ribs in the marinade, coating completely. Cover marinaded short ribs with plastic wrap and refrigerate for 6 to 12 hours3. Preheat pellet grill to 225°F.   Remove plastic wrap from ribs and pull ribs out of marinade. Shake off any excess marinade and dispose of the contents left in the bowl.   Place ribs on grill and cook for about 6-8 hours, until ribs reach an internal temperature of 203°F. Measure using a probe meat thermometer   Once ribs reach temperature, remove from grill and allow to rest for about 20 minutes. Slice, serve, and enjoy!

383. Apple Bourbon Glazed Ham

Servings: 6   Cooking Time: 60 Minutes
Ingredients:
- 1 cup apple jelly
- 2 tablespoons Dijon mustard
- 2 tablespoons bourbon
- 2 tablespoons lemon juice
- ½ teaspoon ground cloves
- 2 cups apple juice
- 1 large ham

Directions:
Fire the   Grill to 500F.   Use maple   wood pellets when cooking. Close the lid and preheat for 15 minutes.   In a small saucepan, combine the apple jelly, mustard, bourbon, lemon juice, cloves, and apple juice. Cook on low heat to melt the apple jelly. Cook for 5 minutes and set aside.   Place the ham in a baking tray and glaze with the reserved mixture.   Place on the grill rack and cook for 60 minutes.   Once the ham is cooked, remove from the grill, and allow to rest for 20 minutes before slicing.   Pour over the remaining glaze.
Nutrition Info: Calories per serving: 283; Protein: 38.7 g; Carbs: 14.7g; Fat: 8g Sugar: 10g

384. Stuffed Peppers

Servings: 6   Cooking Time: 5 Minutes
Ingredients:
- 3 bell peppers, sliced in halves
- 1 pound ground beef, lean
- 1 onion, chopped
- 1/2 tbsp red pepper flakes
- 1/2 tbsp salt
- 1/4 tbsp pepper
- 1/2 tbsp garlic powder
- 1/2 tbsp onion powder
- 1/2 cup white rice
- 15 oz stewed tomatoes
- 8 oz tomato sauce
- 6 cups cabbage, shredded
- 1-1/2 cup water

- 2 cups cheddar cheese

Directions:
Arrange the pepper halves on a baking tray and set aside. Preheat your grill to 325F.   Brown the meat in a large skillet. Add onions, pepper flakes, salt, pepper garlic, and onion and cook until the meat is well cooked.   Add rice, stewed tomatoes, tomato sauce, cabbage, and water. Cover and simmer until the rice is well cooked, the cabbage is tender and there is no water in the rice. Place the cooked beef mixture in the pepper halves and top with cheese.   Place in the grill and cook for 30 minutes.   Serve immediately and enjoy it.
Nutrition Info: Calories: 422 Cal Fat: 22 g Carbohydrates: 24 g   Protein: 34 g Fiber: 5 g

385. Smoked Baby Back Ribs

Servings: 10   Cooking Time: 2 Hours
Ingredients:
- 3 racks baby back ribs
- Salt and pepper to taste

Directions:
Clean the ribs by removing the extra membrane that covers it. Pat dry the ribs with a clean paper towel. Season the baby back ribs with salt and pepper to taste. Allow to rest in the fridge for at least 4 hours before cooking. Once ready to cook, fire the   Grill to 225F.   Use hickory wood pellets when cooking the ribs. Close the lid and preheat for 15 minutes.   Place the ribs on the grill grate and cook for two hours. Carefully flipping the ribs halfway through the cooking time for even cooking.
Nutrition Info: Calories per serving: 1037; Protein: 92.5g; Carbs: 1.4g; Fat: 73.7g Sugar: 0.2g

386. Inexpensive Flank Steak

Servings: 6   Cooking Time: 30 Minutes
Ingredients:
- 1 (2-lb.) beef flank steak
- 2 tbsp. olive oil
- ¼ C. BBQ rub
- 2 tbsp. butter, melted

Directions:
Set the temperature of   Grill to 225 degrees F and preheat with closed lid for 15 minutes.   Coat the steak with oil evenly and season with BBQ rub.   Place the steak onto the grill and cook for about 10-15 minutes per side.   Remove the steak from grill and place onto a cutting board for about 10 minutes before slicing. With a sharp knife, cut the steak into slices across the grain.   Drizzle with melted butter and serve.
Nutrition Info: Calories per serving: 355; Carbohydrates: 0g; Protein: 45.9g; Fat: 17.9g; Sugar: 0g; Sodium: 1607mg; Fiber: 0g

387. Wood Pellet Pulled Pork

Servings: 12   Cooking Time: 12 Hours
Ingredients:

- 8 lb pork shoulder roast, bone-in
- BBQ rub
- 3 cups apple cider, dry hard

Directions:
Fire up the wood pellet grill and set it to smoke. Meanwhile, rub the pork with bbq rub on all sides then place it on the grill grates. cook for 5 hours, flipping it every 1 hour. Increase the heat to 225°F and continue cooking for 3 hours directly on the grate. Transfer the pork to a foil pan and place the apple cider at the bottom of the pan. Cook until the internal temperature reaches 200°F then remove it from the grill. Wrap the pork loosely with foil then let it rest for 1 hour. Remove the fat layer and use forks to shred it. Serve and enjoy.

Nutrition Info: Calories 912, Total fat 65g, Saturated fat 24g, Total Carbs 7g, Net Carbs 7g, Protein 70g, Sugar 6g, Fiber 0g, Sodium: 208mg

388. Tender Flank Steak

Servings: 6   Cooking Time: 10 Minutes
Ingredients:
- ½ C. olive oil
- 1/3 C. fresh lemon juice
- 1/3 C. soy sauce
- ¼ C. brown sugar
- 2 tbsp. Worcestershire sauce
- 5 garlic cloves, minced
- 1 tsp. red chili powder
- 1 tsp. red pepper flakes, crushed
- 2 lb. flank steak

Directions:
In a resealable plastic bag, add all ingredients except for steak and mix well. Place the steak and seal the bag. Shake the bag vigorously to coat well. Refrigerate to marinate overnight. Set the temperature of Grill to 450 degrees F and preheat with closed lid for 15 minutes. Place the steak onto the grill and cook for about 5 minutes per side. Remove the steak from grill and place onto a cutting board for about 10 minutes before slicing. With a sharp knife, cut the steak into slices across the grain.

Nutrition Info: Calories per serving: 482; Carbohydrates: 9.5g; Protein: 43.3g; Fat: 29.6g; Sugar: 7.5g; Sodium: 948mg; Fiber: 0.4g

389. Wood Pellet Grilled Bacon

Servings: 6   Cooking Time: 25 Minutes
Ingredients:
- 1 lb bacon, thickly cut

Directions:
Preheat your wood pellet grill to 375°F. Line a baking sheet with parchment paper then place the bacon on it in a single layer. Close the lid and bake for 20 minutes. Flip over, close the lid, and bake for an additional 5 minutes. Serve with the favorite side and enjoy.

Nutrition Info: Calories 315, Total fat 14g, Saturated fat 10g, Total Carbs 0g, Net Carbs 0g, Protein 9g, Sugar 0g, Fiber 0g, Sodium: 500mg

390. Southern Sugar-glazed Ham

Servings: 12 To 15   Cooking Time: 5 Hours
Ingredients:
- 1 (12- to 15-pound) whole bone-in ham, fully cooked
- ¼ cup yellow mustard
- 1 cup pineapple juice
- ½ cup packed light brown sugar
- 1 teaspoon ground cinnamon
- ½ teaspoon ground cloves

Directions:
Supply your smoker with wood pellets and follow the manufacturer's specific start-up procedure. Preheat, with the lid closed, to 275°F. Trim off the excess fat and skin from the ham, leaving a ¼-inch layer of fat. Put the ham in an aluminum foil–lined roasting pan. On your kitchen stove top, in a medium saucepan over low heat, combine the mustard, pineapple juice, brown sugar, cinnamon, and cloves and simmer for 15 minutes, or until thick and reduced by about half. Baste the ham with half of the pineapple–brown sugar syrup, reserving the rest for basting later in the cook. Place the roasting pan on the grill, close the lid, and smoke for 4 hours. Baste the ham with the remaining pineapple–brown sugar syrup and continue smoking with the lid closed for another hour, or until a meat thermometer inserted in the thickest part of the ham reads 140°F. Remove the ham from the grill, tent with foil, and let rest for 20 minutes before carving.

391. Smoked Tri-tip

Servings: 4   Cooking Time: 5 Hours
Ingredients:
- 1½ pounds tri-tip roast
- Salt
- Freshly ground black pepper
- 2 teaspoons garlic powder
- 2 teaspoons lemon pepper
- ½ cup apple juice

Directions:
Supply your   with wood pellets and follow the start-up procedure. Preheat the grill, with the lid closed, to 180°F. Season the tri-tip roast with salt, pepper, garlic powder, and lemon pepper. Using your hands, work the seasoning into the meat. Place the roast directly on the grill grate and smoke for 4 hours. Pull the tri-tip from the grill and place it on enough aluminum foil to wrap it completely. Increase the grill's temperature to 375°F. Fold in three sides of the foil around the roast and add the apple juice. Fold in the last side, completely enclosing the tri-tip and liquid. Return the wrapped tri-tip to the grill and cook for 45 minutes more. Remove the tri-tip roast from the grill and let it rest for 10 to 15 minutes, before unwrapping, slicing, and serving.

392. Smoked Trip Tip With Java Chophouse

Servings: 4   Cooking Time: 90 Minutes
Ingredients:
- 2 tbsp olive oil
- 2 tbsp java chophouse seasoning
- 3 lb trip tip roast, fat cap and silver skin removed

Directions:
Startup your wood pellet grill and smoker and set the temperature to 225°F.   Rub the roast with olive oil and seasoning then place it on the smoker rack.   Smoke until the internal temperature is 140°F.   Remove the tri-tip from the smoker and let rest for 10 minutes before serving. Enjoy.

Nutrition Info: Calories 270, Total fat 7g, Saturated fat 2g, Total Carbs 0g, Net Carbs 0g, Protein 23g, Sugar 0g, Fiber 0g, Sodium: 47mg, potassium 289mg

393. Thai Beef Skewers

Servings: 6   Cooking Time: 8 Minutes
Ingredients:
- ½ of medium red bell pepper, destemmed, cored, cut into a ¼-inch piece
- ½ of beef sirloin, fat trimmed
- ½ cup salted peanuts, roasted, chopped
- For the Marinade:
- 1 teaspoon minced garlic
- 1 tablespoon grated ginger
- 1 lime, juiced
- 1 teaspoon ground black pepper
- 1 tablespoon sugar
- 1/4 cup soy sauce
- 1/4 cup olive oil

Directions:
Prepare the marinade and for this, take a small bowl, place all of its ingredients in it, whisk until combined, and then pour it into a large plastic bag.   Cut into beef sirloin 1-1/4-inch dice, add to the plastic bag containing marinade, seal the bag, turn it upside down to coat beef pieces with the marinade and let it marinate for a minimum of 2 hours in the refrigerator.   When ready to cook, switch on the   grill, fill the grill hopper with cherry flavored wood pellets, power the grill on by using the control panel, select 'smoke' on the temperature dial, or set the temperature to 425 degrees F and let it preheat for a minimum of 5 minutes.   Meanwhile, remove beef pieces from the marinade and then thread onto skewers. When the grill has preheated, open the lid, place prepared skewers on the grill grate, shut the grill, and smoke for 4 minutes per side until done.   When done, transfer skewers to a dish, sprinkle with peanuts and red pepper, and then serve.

Nutrition Info: Calories: 124 Cal ;Fat: 5.5 g ;Carbs: 1.7 g ;Protein: 15.6 g ;Fiber: 0 g

394. Smoked Lamb Leg With Salsa Verde

Servings: 6   Cooking Time: 3 Hours
Ingredients:
- 2 tablespoons oil
- 1 whole leg of lamb, fat trimmed and cut into chunks
- Salt to taste
- 6 cloves green garlic, unpeeled
- 1-pound tomatillos, husked and washed
- 1 small yellow onion, quartered
- 5 whole serrano chili peppers
- 1 tablespoon capers, drained
- ¼ cup cilantro, finely chopped
- ½ teaspoon sugar
- 1 cup chicken broth
- 3 tablespoons lime juice, freshly squeezed

Directions:
Fire the   Grill to 500F. Use desired   wood pellets when cooking. Close the lid and preheat for 15 minutes. Place a Dutch oven on the grill grate and add oil.   Put the lamb in the Dutch oven and season with salt to taste. Stir once then close the lid.   Place the garlic, tomatillos, onion, serrano peppers, and capers in a parchment-lined baking tray.   Season with salt to taste and drizzle with olive oil.   Place in the grill and cook for 15 minutes. Remove the vegetables from the grill and transfer to a blender. Add cilantro and sugar. Season with more salt if needed. Pulse until smooth then set aside.   Pour the mixture into the Dutch oven and add in chicken broth and lime juice.   Allow to cook for 3 hours.

Nutrition Info: Calories per serving: 430;
Protein: 56.4g; Carbs: 7.8g; Fat: 18.4g Sugar: 3.9g

395. Wood Pellet Grilled Lamb With Brown Sugar Glaze

Servings: 4   Cooking Time: 10 Minutes
Ingredients:
- 1/4 cup brown sugar
- 2 tbsp ginger, ground
- 2 tbsp tarragon, dried
- 1 tbs cinnamon, ground
- 1 tbsp black pepper, ground
- 1 tbsp garlic powder
- 1/2 tbsp salt
- 4 lamb chops

Directions:
In a mixing bowl, mix sugar, ginger, dried tarragon, cinnamon, black pepper, garlic, and salt.   Rub the lamb chops with the seasoning and place it on a plate.refrigerate for an hour to marinate.   Preheat the grill to high heat then brush the grill grate with oil. Arrange the lamb chops on the grill grate in a single layer and cook for 5 minutes on each side.   Serve and enjoy.

Nutrition Info: Calories 241, Total fat 13.1g, Saturated fat 6g, Total Carbs 15.8g, Net Carbs 15.1g, Protein 14.6g, Sugar 14g, Fiber 0.7g, Sodium: 339mg,

396. Bbq Brown Sugar Bacon

Servings: 3   Cooking Time: 30 Minutes
Ingredients:
- ½ cup brown sugar

- 1 tablespoon fennel, ground
- 2 teaspoons salt
- 1 teaspoon black pepper
- 1-pound pork belly, sliced thinly into bacon

Directions:
Place all ingredients in a bowl and mix until well combined. Allow seasoned pork to rest in the fridge for at least 3 hours.   When ready to cook, fire the Grill to 255F. Use maple wood pellets when cooking. Close the lid and preheat for 15 minutes.   Place the bacon on the grill grate and close the lid. Smoke for 20 to 30 minutes.

Nutrition Info: Calories per serving: 331 ;
Protein: 26.2g; Carbs: 39.7g; Fat: 8.5g Sugar: 26.7g

397. Cowboy Steak

Servings: 4   Cooking Time: 1 Hour

Ingredients:
- 2.5 lb. cowboy cut steaks
- Salt to taste
- Beef rub
- 1/4 cup olive oil
- 2 tablespoons fresh mint leaves, chopped
- ½ cup parsley, chopped
- 1 clove garlic, crushed and minced
- 1 tablespoon lemon juice
- 1 tablespoon lemon zest
- Salt and pepper to taste

Directions:
Season the steak with the salt and dry rub.   Preheat the wood pellet grill to 225 degrees F for 10 minutes while the lid is closed.   Grill the steaks for 45 minutes, flipping once or twice.   Increase temperature to 450 degrees F.   Put the steaks back to the grill. Cook for 5 minutes per side.   In a bowl, mix the remaining ingredients.   Serve steaks with the parsley mixture.
Tips: Let steak rest for 10 minutes before putting it back to the grill for the second round of cooking.

398. Herby Lamb Chops

Servings: 4   Cooking Time: 2 Hours

Ingredients:
- 8 lamb chops, each about ¾-inch thick, fat trimmed
- For the Marinade:
- 1 teaspoon minced garlic
- Salt as needed
- 1 tablespoon dried rosemary
- Ground black pepper as needed
- ½ tablespoon dried thyme
- 3 tablespoons balsamic vinegar
- 1 tablespoon Dijon mustard
- ½ cup olive oil

Directions:
Prepare the marinade and for this, take a small bowl, place all of its ingredients in it and stir until well combined.   Place lamb chops in a large plastic bag, pour in marinade, seal the bag, turn it upside down to coat lamb chops with the marinade and let it marinate

for a minimum of 4 hours in the refrigerator.   When ready to cook, switch on the   grill, fill the grill hopper with flavored wood pellets, power the grill on by using the control panel, select 'smoke' on the temperature dial, or set the temperature to 450 degrees F and let it preheat for a minimum of 5 minutes.   Meanwhile, remove lamb chops from the refrigerator and bring them to room temperature.   When the grill has preheated, open the lid, place lamb chops on the grill grate, shut the grill and smoke for 5 minutes per side until seared. When done, transfer lamb chops to a dish, let them rest for 5 minutes and then serve.

Nutrition Info: Calories: 280 Cal ;Fat: 12.3 g ;Carbs: 8.3 g ;Protein: 32.7 g ;Fiber: 1.2 g

399. Lamb Chops

Servings: 8   Cooking Time: 10 Minutes

Ingredients:
- For the Lamb:
- 16 lamb chops, fat trimmed
- 2 tablespoons Greek Freak seasoning
- For the Mint Sauce:
- 1 tablespoon chopped parsley
- 12 cloves of garlic, peeled
- 1 tablespoon chopped mint
- 1/4 teaspoon dried oregano
- 1 teaspoon salt
- 1/4 teaspoon ground black pepper
- 3/4 cup lemon juice
- 1 cup olive oil

Directions:
Prepare the mint sauce and for this, place all of its ingredients in a food processor and then pulse for 1 minute until smooth.   Pour 1/3 cup of the mint sauce into a plastic bag, add lamb chops in it, seal the bag, turn it upside to coat lamb chops with the sauce and then let them marinate for a minimum of 30 minutes in the refrigerator.   When ready to cook, switch on the   grill, fill the grill hopper with apple-flavored wood pellets, power the grill on by using the control panel, select 'smoke' on the temperature dial, or set the temperature to 450 degrees F and let it preheat for a minimum of 15 minutes.   Meanwhile, remove lamb chops from the marinade and then season with Greek seasoning. When the grill has preheated, open the lid, place lamb chops on the grill grate, shut the grill and smoke for 4 to 5 minutes per side until cooked to the desired level. When done, transfer lamb chops to a dish and then serve.

Nutrition Info: Calories: 362 Cal ;Fat: 26 g ;Carbs: 0 g ;Protein: 31 g ;Fiber: 0 g

400. Wood Pellet Grilled Aussie Leg Of Lamb Roast

Servings: 8   Cooking Time: 2 Hours

Ingredients:
- 5 lb Aussie leg of lamb, boneless
- Smoked Paprika Rub
- 1 tbsp raw sugar

- 1 tbsp kosher salt
- 1 tbsp black pepper
- 1 tbsp smoked paprika
- 1 tbsp garlic powder
- 1 tbsp rosemary, dried
- 1 tbsp onion powder
- 1tbsp cumin
- 1/2 tbsp cayenne pepper
- Roasted Carrots
- 1 bunch rainbow carrots
- Olive oil
- Salt
- pepper

Directions:
Heat the wood pellet grill to 375 F.   Trim any excess fat from the lamb.   Combine all the rub ingredients and rub all over the lamb. Place the lamb on the grill and smoke for 2 hours.   Toss the carrots in oil, salt, and pepper then add to the grill after the lamb has cooked for 1-1/2 hour.   Cook until the roast internal temperature reaches 135 F. Remove the lamb from the grill and cover with foil. Let rest for 30 minutes.   Remove the carrots from the grill once soft and serve with the lamb. Enjoy.

Nutrition Info: Calories 257, Total fat 8g, Saturated fat 2g, Total Carbs 6g, Net Carbs 5g, Protein 37g, Sugar 3g, Fiber 1g, Sodium: 431mg, Potassium 666mg

OTHER FAVORITE RECIPES

401. Prosciutto-wrapped Melon

Servings: 8   Cooking Time: 25 Minutes
Ingredients:
- 1ripe cantaloupe
- Salt and pepper
- 16thin slices prosciutto

Directions:
Start the coals or heat a gas grill for medium direct cooking. Make sure the grates are clean.   Cut the cantaloupe in half lengthwise and scoop out all the seeds. Cut each half into 8 wedges, then cut away the rind from each wedge. Sprinkle with salt and pepper and wrap each wedge with a slice of prosciutto, covering as much of the cantaloupe as possible.   Put the wedges on the grill directly over the fire. Close the lid and cook, turning once, until the prosciutto shrivels, browns, and crisps in places, 2 to 3 minutes per side. Serve hot or at room temperature.
Nutrition Info: Calories: 118.3 Fats: 5.4 g Cholesterol: 0 mg Carbohydrates: 12.5 g Fiber: 1.1 g Sugars: 0 g Proteins: 6.7 g

402. Eastern North-carolina Bbq Sauce

Servings: 1 Cup   Cooking Time: 5 Minutes
Ingredients:
- ½ cup white vinegar
- ½ cup cider vinegar
- ½ tablespoon sugar
- ½ tablespoon crushed red pepper flakes
- ½ tablespoon Tabasco sauce
- Salt and freshly cracked black pepper to taste

Directions:
Whisk ingredients together in a bowl. Drizzle on barbecued meat. Covered, sauce will keep about 2 months.

403. Cold Hot Smoked Salmon

Servings: 4   Cooking Time: 8 Hours
Ingredients:
- 5 pound of fresh sockeye (red) salmon fillets
- For trout Brine
- 4 cups of filtered water
- 1 cup of soy sauce
- ½ a cup of pickling kosher salt
- ½ a cup of brown sugar
- 2 tablespoon of garlic powder
- 2 tablespoon of onion powder
- 1 teaspoon of cayenne pepper

Directions:
Combine all of the ingredients listed under trout brine in two different 1-gallon bags. Store it in your fridge. Cut up the Salmon fillets into 3-4-inch pieces. Place your salmon pieces into your 1-gallon container of trout brine and let it keep in your fridge for 8 hours.   Rotate the Salmon and pat them dry using a kitchen towel for 8 hours Configure your pellet smoker for indirect cooking. Remove your salmon pieces of from your fridge Preheat your smoker to a temperature of 180 degrees Fahrenheit Once a cold smoke at 70 degrees Fahrenheit starts smoke your fillets   Keep smoking it until the internal temperature reaches 145 degrees Fahrenheit.   Remove the Salmon from your smoker and let it rest for 10 minutes
Nutrition Info: Calories: 849 Cal Fat: 45 g Carbohydrates: 51 g   Protein: 46 g Fiber: 0 g

404. Stuffed Burgers

Servings: 6   Cooking Time: 15 Minutes
Ingredients:
- 3 lb ground beef
- 1/2 tbsp onion powder
- 1/4 tbsp garlic powder
- 1 tbsp salt
- 1/2 tbsp pepper
- 1-1/2 cups Colby jack cheese, shredded
- Johnny's seasoning salt
- 6 slices Colby Jack cheese

Directions:
Preheat your   to 375F.   Mix beef, onion powder, garlic powder, salt, and pepper until well combined. Make 12 patties.   Place cheese on the burger patty and cover with another patty then seal the edges.   Season with salt, then place the patties on the grill. Cook the patties on the grill grate for 8 minutes, flip the patties and cook for additional 5 minutes.   Place a slice of cheese on each patty and grill with the lid closed to melt the cheese.   Remove the patties from the   and let rest for 10 minutes. Serve and enjoy with a toasted bun.
Nutrition Info: Calories 463, Total fat 29g, Saturated fat 18g, Total carbs 1g, Net carbs 1g Protein 67g, Sugars 2g, Fiber 0g, Sodium 590mg

405. Bbq Elk Short Ribs

Servings: 6   Cooking Time: 1 Hour
Ingredients:
- 1/2 pound green beans
- 3 pounds elk short ribs
- 1/2 pound chanterelle mushrooms
- 6 ounces rib rub
- Salt as needed
- Ground black pepper as needed
- 4 tablespoons unsalted butter

Directions:
Switch on the   grill, fill the grill hopper with cherry flavored wood pellets, power the grill on by using the control panel, select 'smoke' on the temperature dial, or set the temperature to 275 degrees F and let it preheat for a minimum of 15 minutes.   Meanwhile, prepare the ribs, and for this, season them with salt and rib rub until

well coated.   When the grill has preheated, open the lid, place ribs on the grill grate rib-side down, shut the grill and smoke for 30 minutes.   Then wrap ribs in foil in the double layer, return to the grill grate and continue smoking 15 minutes or until the internal temperature reaches 125 degrees.   When done, transfer ribs to a dish and let them rest until required.   Change the smoking temperature to 450 degrees F, shut with lid, and let it preheat for 15 minutes.   Then place a skillet pan on the grill grate and when hot, add butter and when it melts, add mushrooms and beans, toss until mixed, shut with lid, and cook for 15 minutes until vegetables have turned tender and golden brown.   Serve grilled vegetables with elk ribs.

Nutrition Info: Calories: 393 Cal ;Fat: 16.6 g ;Carbs: 25 g ;Protein: 36 g ;Fiber: 0.9 g

406. Roasted Lamb

Servings: 8   Cooking Time: 1 Hour And 30 Minutes
Ingredients:
- 1 leg of lamb
- 8 cloves garlic, minced
- 1 sprig oregano, chopped
- 2 sprigs rosemary, chopped
- 6 tablespoons olive oil
- 2 tablespoons lemon juice
- Salt and pepper to taste

Directions:
Make slits on the lamb leg.   Combine the garlic and herbs.   Mash to form a paste.   Stuff mixture inside the slits.   Add the lamb leg to a roasting pan.   Drizzle it with olive oil and lemon juice.   Cover with foil and refrigerate for 10 hours.   When ready to cook, sprinkle lamb with salt and pepper.   Set the   wood pellet grill to 400 degrees F.   Preheat for 15 minutes while the lid is closed.   Open the lid and let it establish fire for 5 minutes.   Roast the leg of lamb for 30 minutes. Reduce temperature to 350 degrees F and cook for 1 hour. Let rest before slicing and serving.   Tips: You can also use a food processor to create a paste from the garlic and herbs.

407. Smoked Italian Meatballs

Servings: 6   Cooking Time: 1 Hour 5 Minutes;
Ingredients:
- 2 lb beef, ground
- 2 slices white bread
- 1/2 cup whole milk
- 1 tbsp salt
- 1/2 tbsp onion powder
- 1/2 tbsp minced garlic
- 2 tbsp Italian seasoning
- 1/4 tbsp black pepper

Directions:
In a mixing bowl, mix all the ingredients until well combined using your hands. Turn on your   and set it to smoke then line a baking sheet with parchment paper. Roll golf size meatballs using your hands .and place them

on the baking dish. Place the baking dish in the   and smoke for 35 minutes.   Increase the   heat to 325F and cook for 30 more minutes or until the internal temperature reaches 160F.   Serve when hot

Nutrition Info: Calories 453, Total fat 27g, Saturated fat 10g, Total carbs 7g, Net carbs 7g Protein 0g, Sugars 2g, Fiber 0g, Sodium 550mg

408. White Bbq Sauce

Servings: 3 Cups   Cooking Time: 10 Minutes
Ingredients:
- 1 ½ cups mayonnaise
- ⅓ cup plus 2 tablespoons apple-cider vinegar
- 2 tablespoons lemon juice
- 2 tablespoons prepared horseradish
- 1 teaspoon mustard powder
- Kosher salt and freshly ground black pepper, to taste
- cayenne pepper, to taste

Directions:
Combine the mayonnaise, vinegar, lemon juice, horseradish and mustard powder in a medium nonreactive bowl, and whisk until smooth.   Add salt, pepper and cayenne to taste. Brush on grilled or roasted chicken during the end of the cooking process, and pass remaining sauce at the table.

409. Lamb Shanks, Smoke-braised

Servings: 2   Cooking Time: 5 Hours 20 Minutes
Ingredients:
- 1/2 cup of brown sugar
- 2 cups of water
- 4 strips of orange
- 2 cinnamon sticks
- 3 whole of star anise
- 1/2 cup of soy sauce
- 2 shank of lamb
- 1/2 cup of rice wine
- 3 Tbsp of sesame oil, Asian

Directions:
Put the lamb shank on an aluminum foil paper.   In a bowl, mix the sesame oil, water, soy sauce, and brown sugar in a bowl until the sugar dissolves. Add the cinnamon stick, orange zest, and star anise to the bowl. Pour the mixture on the lamb.   Preheat the grill for 15 minutes at 250°F. Use alder wood pellets   Place the lamb shank on the cooking grates with the foil. Smoke the lamb for 5 hours, until it is brown.   Remove the lamb from the smoker and place it on a board to trim off excess fat. Serve immediately.

Nutrition Info: Per Serving: Calories: 255kcal, Carbs: 46g, Fat: 36g, Protein: 34.1g.

410. Pan-seared Pork Tenderloin With Apple Mashed Potatoes

Servings: 6   Cooking Time: 20 Minutes

Ingredients:
- 2 pork tenderloin
- medium potatoes (peeled and sliced)
- 3 Tbsp unsalted butter
- 1/2 cup of heavy cream
- 2 Tbsp Olive oil
- 1-1/2 Tbsp Pepper
- 1-1/2 Tbsp Salt.
- 2 apple (cored and sliced)

Directions:
Preheat the wood pellet smoker-grill for direct cooking at 300 F using any pellet.   Season the pork with salt and pepper, then roast meat for 20 minutes.   Increase the temperature of the grill to High, then place an iron skillet on the grates, and add 1 Tbsp butter and oil. Cook until the butter becomes brown, make sure it does not burn. Place the tenderloin and cook for 4 minutes per side or until it is brown, transfer to a baking sheet and bake for 10 minutes.   Rearrange the grill for indirect cooking at 300 F   Place a pot over the cooking grid and fill it with water. Add potatoes and allow to boil, reduce the heat and simmer for 8 minutes or until soft. Drain the water Pour the potatoes into a food processor, add cream and butter. Puree the mixture, add the apples and puree until they are finely chopped. Season with salt and pepper and serve with the pork.

Nutrition Info: Per Serving: Calories: 477kcal, Carbs: 26.9g, Fat: 24.5g, Protein: 46.5g

411. Baked Wild Sockeye Salmon

Servings: 6   Cooking Time: 45 Minutes
Ingredients:
- 6 sockeye salmon fillets
- 3/4 tsp Old bay seasoning
- 1/2 tsp Seafood seasoning.

Directions:
Set the wood pellet smoker-grill to indirect cooking at 400 F   Rinse the fillet and pat dry with a paper towel. Add the seasoning, then rub all over the fillets. Arrange fillets in a baking dish with the skin facing down, then transfer the dish to the cooking grid. Cover grill and bake for 15-20 minutes or until fillets begin to flake. Serve.

Nutrition Info: Per Serving: Calories: 294kcal, Carbs: 10g, Fat:1g, Protein: 26g

412. Rib Roast And Yorkshire Pudding With Bacon And Rosemary Jus

Servings: 10   Cooking Time: 45 Minutes
Ingredients:
- 1 Tbsp of black pepper
- 1 bacon with rosemary jus
- 3 Tbsp of thyme, preferably fresh leaves
- 6 cloves of garlic, already peeled
- 2-1/2 Tbsp of salt
- 2-1/2 Tbsp of olive oil
- 1 of 5-bone of rib-eye roast, standing
- 1 scallion with parmesan Yorkshire pudding

Directions:
Put garlic inside a running food processor. Scrape it into a bowl, mix with pepper, salt, thyme, and oil until a paste is formed.   Preheat the grill for direct cooking at 350°F. Use mesquite wood pellets for a distinctive, strong woody taste.   Press the herb mixture into the sliced ribs. Put the ribs in the roasting pan and roast both sides for 20 minutes or until internal temperature reads 145°F. Allow the ribs to rest for 10 minutes before serving. After then, serve with Yorkshire pudding.

Nutrition Info: Per Serving: Calories: 250kcal, Protein: 25.6g, Carbs: 33g, Fat: 25.5g.

413. Honey Dipping Sauce

Servings: 4   Cooking Time: 10 Minutes
Ingredients:
- 5 tablespoons unsalted butter
- 8 tablespoons kimchi paste
- 2 tablespoons honey
- 1 tsp sesame seeds

Directions:
In a blender place all ingredients and blend until smooth Pour sauce in a bowl and serve

414. Spiced Nuts

Servings: 32   Cooking Time: 20 Minutes
Ingredients:
- 1teaspoon dried rosemary
- 1/8 teaspoon cayenne pepper
- 1/8 teaspoon ground black pepper
- ½ teaspoon salt or to taste
- ½ teaspoon ground cuminutes
- 1tablespoon olive oil
- 2tablespoon maple syrup
- 2/3 cup raw and unsalted cashew nuts
- 2/3 cup raw and unsalted pecans
- 2/3 cup raw and unsalted walnuts

Directions:
Start your grill on smoke mode, leaving the lid open for 5 minutes, until the fire starts.   Close the grill lid and preheat the grill to 350°F.   In a large bowl, combine all the ingredients except the dried rosemary. Mix thoroughly until the ingredients are evenly mixed, and all nuts are coated with spices.   Spread the spiced nuts on a baking sheet.   Place the baking sheet on the grill and roast the nuts for 20 to 25 minutes.   Remove the nuts from heat.   Sprinkle the dried rosemary on the nuts and stir to mix.   Leave the nuts to cool for a few minutes.   Serve and enjoy.

Nutrition Info: Calories: 64 Total Fat: 5.8 g Saturated Fat: 0.4 g Cholesterol: 0 mg Sodium: 35 mg Total Carbohydrate 2.2 g Dietary Fiber 0.6 g Total Sugars: 0.8 g Protein: 1.3 g

415. Turkey Sandwich

Servings: 4   Cooking Time: 20 Minutes

Ingredients:
- 8 bread slices
- 1 cup gravy
- 2 cups turkey, cooked and shredded

Directions:
Set your wood pellet grill to smoke.   Preheat it to 400 degrees F.   Place a grill mat on top of the grates. Add the turkey on top of the mat.   Cook for 10 minutes. Toast the bread in the flame broiler.   Top the bread with the gravy and shredded turkey.

Nutrition Info: Calories: 280 Fat: 3.5 g Cholesterol: 20 mg Carbohydrates: 46 g Fiber: 5 g Sugars: 7 g Protein: 18 g

416. Pork And Portobello Burgers

Servings: 4   Cooking Time: 30 Minutes

Ingredients:
- 1 pound ground pork
- 1 tablespoon minced garlic
- 1 teaspoon minced fresh rosemary, fennel seed or parsley
- Salt and ground black pepper
- 4 large portobello mushroom caps, stems removed
- Olive oil
- 4 burger buns
- Any burger fixings you like

Directions:
Combine the ground pork, garlic, rosemary and a sprinkle of salt and pepper. Use a spoon to lightly scrape away the gills of the mushrooms and hollow them slightly. Drizzle the mushrooms (inside and out) with olive oil and sprinkle with salt and pepper. Press 1/4 of the mixture into each of the hollow sides of the mushrooms; you want the meat to spread all the way across the width of the mushrooms. They should look like burgers.   Grill the burgers, meat side down, until the pork is well browned, 4 to 6 minutes. Flip and cook until the top side of the mushrooms are browned and the mushrooms are tender, another 6 to 8 minutes. If you like, use an instant-read thermometer to check the interior temperature of the pork, which should be a minimum of 145 degrees.   Serve the burgers on buns (toasted, if you like) with any fixings you like.

417. Bourbon Braised Beef Short Ribs

Servings: 6   Cooking Time: 3 Hours 15 Minutes

Ingredients:
- 2 Tbsp Worcestershire sauce
- 3 Tbsp soy sauce
- 2 Tbsp bourbon
- 1/2 cup Dijon mustard
- 1 cup beef stock
- 12   beef short ribs

Directions:
Preheat wood pellet smoker-grill to 250°F, with the lid closed for about 15 minutes   Mix the Worcestershire sauce, mustard, and molasses.   Brush sauce on each side of the rib.   Prepare the mop sauce by mixing the soy sauce, beef stock, and bourbon in a food-safe plastic spray bottle.   Arrange the ribs directly on the grill and braise for 2 hours, until an internal temperature of 165°F is reached. Spray the mop sauce over the rib occasionally for tender perfection.   Remove rib from the grill and place on an aluminum foil. Pour remaining mop sauce over the ribs and wrap the foil over the ribs.   Transfer foil enclosed rib for direct cooking to the grill grate. Braise the ribs until the Instant read thermometer reads a temperature of 195°F, about one hour.   Remove foil enclosed rib from grill and place on a platter to rest for 15 minutes   Take out ribs from foil and serve.

Nutrition Info: Per Serving: Calories: 591kcal, Carbs: 78g,   Fat: 13g, Protein: 8g

418. Roasted Ham

Servings: 12   Cooking Time: 6 Hours

Ingredients:
- 2 quarts water
- 1/2 cup quick home meat cure
- 1/2 cup kosher salt
- 3/4 cup brown sugar
- 1 tablespoon pork rub
- 1 teaspoon whole cloves
- 10 lb. fresh ham
- 1 teaspoon whole cloves
- 1/4 cup pure maple syrup
- 2 cup apple juice

Directions:
In a large container, pour in the water and add the meat cure, salt, sugar, pork rub and whole cloves.   Mix well. Soak the ham in the brine.   Cover and refrigerate for 1 day.   Rinse ham with water and dry with paper towels. Score the ham with crosshatch pattern.   Insert remaining cloves into the ham.   Season ham with the pork rub.   Add ham to a roasting pan.   Smoke the ham in the   wood pellet grill for 2 hours at 180 degrees F.   Make the glaze by mixing the maple syrup and apple juice.   Brush the ham with this mixture. Increase heat to 300 degrees F.   Roast for 4 hours. Tips: You can also inject the brine into the ham.

419. Hot Sauce With Cilantro

Servings: 4   Cooking Time: 10 Minutes

Ingredients:
- ½ tsp coriander
- ½ tsp cumin seeds
- ¼ tsp black pepper
- 2 green cardamom pods
- 2 garlic cloves
- 1 tsp salt
- 1 oz. parsley
- 2 tablespoons olive oil

Directions:
In a blender place all ingredients and blend until smooth Pour sauce in a bowl and serve

420. Smoky Caramelized Onions On The Pellet Grill

Servings: 4   Cooking Time: 1 Hour
Ingredients:
- 5 large sliced onions
- 1/2 cup fat of your choice
- Pinch of Sea salt

Directions:
Place all the ingredients into a pan. For a deep rich brown caramelized onion, cook them off for about 1hour on a stovetop.   Keep the grill temperatures not higher than 250 - 275F.   Now transfer the pan into the grill. Cook for about 1-1½ hours until brown. Check and stir with a spoon, wooden, after every 15 minutes. Make sure not to run out of pellets.   Now remove from the grill and season with more salt if necessary.   Serve immediately or place in a refrigerator for up to 1 week.
Nutrition Info: Calories: 286 Total Fat: 25.8 g Saturated Fat: 10.3 g Total Carbs: 12.8 g Net Carbs: 9.8 g Protein: 1.5 g Sugars: 5.8 g Fiber: 3 g Sodium: 6 mg

421. Grilled Watermelon

Servings: 2-3   Cooking Time: 2 Minutes
Ingredients:
- 6watermelon slices, each measuring 3 inches across and 1-inch thick
- 2tablespoons honey

Directions:
Put the grill grate inside the hood and close the unit. Set temperature to the max and set the timer to 2 minutes.   Stop the unit as it is preheated.   Now brush the watermelon slices with honey.   Grease the grill grate with oil spray.   Place the watermelon slices on the grill grate.   Close the hood and grill for 2 minutes without flipping it.   Once done, take out watermelon slices and serve immediately.
Nutrition Info: Calories: 322 Total Fat: 1.1g Saturated Fat: 0.6g Cholesterol: 0mg Sodium: 12mg Total Carbohydrate: 81.8g Dietary Fiber 3.4g Total Sugars: 69.9g Protein: 5.1g.

422. Potluck Favorite Baked Beans

Servings: 10   Cooking Time: 3 Hours 5 Minutes
Ingredients:
- 1 tbsp. butter
- ½ of red bell pepper, seeded and chopped
- ½ of medium onion, chopped
- 2 jalapeño peppers, chopped
- 2 (28-oz.) cans baked beans, rinsed and drained
- 8 oz. pineapple chunks, drained
- 1 C. BBQ sauce
- 1 C. brown sugar
- 1 tbsp. ground mustard

Directions:
Set the temperature of   Grill to 220-250 degrees F and preheat with closed lid for 15 minutes.   In a non-stick skillet, melt butter over medium heat and sauté the bell peppers, onion and jalapeño peppers for about 4-5 minutes.   Remove from heat and transfer the pepper mixture into a bowl.   Add remaining ingredients and stir to combine.   Transfer the mixture into a Dutch oven.   Place the Dutch oven onto the grill and cook for about 2½-3 hours.   Remove from grill and serve hot.
Nutrition Info: Calories per serving: 364; Carbohydrates: 61.4g; Protein: 9.4g; Fat: 9.8g; Sugar: 23.5g; Sodium: 1036mg; Fiber: 9.7g

423. Beef Pot Roast

Servings: 6   Cooking Time: 3 Hours 10 Minutes
Ingredients:
- 3 cup beef stock
- 1 cup carrots, chopped
- 1 Tbsp garlic, minced
- 1/4 cup softened butter
- 1 Tsp ground black pepper
- 2 red onions, chopped
- 4lb chuck roast
- 1 Tbsp kosher salt
- 1Tbsp sage, chopped
- 1/2 cup red wine

Directions:
Preheat   Grill & Smoker to 300ºF with the cover of the grill closed for 10 minutes.   In a stockpot, put in red wine, beef stock, butter, garlic, carrot, red onion, sage, and chuck roast—season with pepper and salt. Stir the contents and cover the pot.   Transfer stockpot to the preheated grill; close the grill lid and leave to cook for 3 hours, until the roast reaches an internal temperature of 203ºF.   Serve.
Nutrition Info: Per Serving: Calories: 487kcal, Carbs: 19g, Fat: 17g, Protein: 6.0g

424. Bison Burgers

Servings: 6   Cooking Time: 17 To 19 Minutes
Ingredients:
- 2 pounds ground bison
- 2 tablespoons steak seasoning
- 4 tablespoons (½ stick) unsalted butter, cut into pieces
- 1 large onion, finely minced
- 6 slices Swiss cheese
- 6 ciabatta buns, split
- Sweet and Spicy Jalapeño Relish, for serving
- Lettuce and sliced tomatoes, for serving

Directions:
Supply your smoker with wood pellets and follow the manufacturer's specific start-up procedure. Preheat, with the lid closed, to 425°F.   In a large bowl, combine the ground bison and steak seasoning until well blended. Shape the meat mixture into 6 patties and make a thumb indentation in the center of each. Set aside.   Place a rimmed baking sheet on the grill and add the butter and onion. Sauté for 5 minutes, or until the onion is translucent. Top with the bison burger patties,

indention-side down.   Close the lid and smoke for 6 to 7 minutes, then flip the burgers and smother them in the sautéed onion. Close the lid again and continue smoking for 6 to 7 minutes. During the last few minutes of cooking, top each burger with a slice of Swiss cheese. For safe consumption, the internal temperature should reach between 140°F (medium) and 160°F (well-done). Lightly toast the ciabatta buns, split-side down, on one side of the smoker.   Serve the onion-smothered cheeseburgers on the toasted buns with jalapeño relish, lettuce, and tomato—or whatever toppings you like.

425. Grilled Tuna Burger With Ginger Mayonnaise

Servings: 4   Cooking Time: 20 Minutes
Ingredients:
- 1 Tbsp of sesame oil, optional
- 4 Tbsp of ginger, optional
- 4 hamburger buns
- Black pepper, freshly ground
- 2 Tbsp and 1 tsp of soy sauce
- 4 of 5 ounces of tuna steak
- Natural oil
- 1/2 cup of mayonnaise

Directions:
Set the grill for direct cooking at 300°F. Use maple pellets for a robust woody taste.   Rub soy sauce on the tuna steak and season with pepper.   In another bowl, prepare a rub by mixing the ginger, mayonnaise, 1 tsp of soy sauce, and sesame oil.   With a brush, apply the rub on the tuna steak then grill for 10 minutes before flipping. Grill the other side for another 10 minutes.   Serve immediately with fish between buns. Add mayonnaise and ginger as layers.
Nutrition Info: Per Serving: Calories: 220kcal, Protein: 21.5g, Fat: 16g, Carbs: 23g.

426. Cajun Shrimp

Servings: 4   Cooking Time: 10 Minutes
Ingredients:
- 4 tablespoon olive oil
- 1 tablespoon lemon juice
- 2 cloves garlic, minced
- 1 tablespoon Cajun rub
- Salt to taste
- 2 lb. shrimp, peeled and deveined

Directions:
Mix all the ingredients in a bowl.   Cover the bowl and refrigerate for 3 hours.   Set the   grill to high and preheat for 15 minutes while the lid is closed.   Thread the shrimp onto skewers.   Grill the shrimp for 4 minutes per side.   Tips: If using wooden skewers, soak first in water for 15 minutes before using.

427. Rosemary Cheese Bread

Servings: 30   Cooking Time: 12 Minutes

Ingredients:
- 1½ cup sunflower seeds
- ½ tsp sea salt
- 1egg
- 1tsp fresh rosemary (finely chopped)
- 2tsp xanthan gum
- 2tbsp cream cheese
- 2cups grated mozzarella

Directions:
Preheat the grill to 400°F with the lid closed for 15 minutes.   Toss the sunflower seeds into a powerful blender and blend until it smooth and flour-like. Transfer the sunflower seed flour into a mixing bowl and add the rosemary and xanthan gum. Mix and set aside. Melt the cheese in a microwave. To do this, combine the cream cheese and mozzarella cheese in a microwave-safe dish.   Place the microwave-safe dish in the grill and heat the cheese on high for 1 minute.   Bring out the dish and stir. Place the dish in the grill and heat for 30 seconds. Bring out the dish and stir until smooth. Pour the melted cheese into a large mixing bowl.   Add the sunflower flour mixture to the melted cheese and stir the ingredients are well combined.   Add the salt and egg and mix thoroughly to form a smooth dough. Measure out equal pieces of the dough and roll into sticks. Grease a baking sheet with oil and arrange the breadsticks into the baking sheet in a single layer.   Use the back of a knife or metal spoon to make lines on the breadsticks.   Place the baking sheet on the grill and make for about 12 minutes or until the breadsticks turn golden brown.   Remove the baking sheet from the grill and let the breadsticks cool for a few minutes.   Serve.
Nutrition Info: Calories: 23 Total Fat: 1.9 g Saturated Fat: 0.5 g Cholesterol: 7 mg Sodium: 47 mg Total Carbohydrate: 0.6 g Dietary Fiber: 0.2 g Total Sugars: 0.1 g Protein: 1.2 g

428. beef Pot Pie

Servings: 8   Cooking Time: 60 Minutes
Ingredients:
- 1 pie crust
- Pot Pie
- 2 cups potatoes, diced
- 3 cups leftover pot roast
- 1 cup corn
- 1 cup carrots
- 1/2 cup peas
- 1/2 cup green beans
- Gravy
- 1/4 cup butter +2 tbsp
- 1/4 cup flour
- 3 cups beef broth
- 1/4 tbsp sherry
- 1/2 tbsp onion powder
- 1/8 tbsp garlic powder
- 1/4 thyme
- Egg Wash
- 1 egg yolk
- 1 tbsp water

Directions:

Preheat your to 350F. Take the potatoes and drizzle with some oil then sprinkle with salt. Microwave them for 4 minutes. Place the pot pie ingredients in a cast iron pan. Melt butter in a nonstick skillet, then whisk in flour until there are no lumps. Stir cook the mixture for 7 minutes over medium heat. Whisk in broth, sherry, onion powder, garlic powder, and thyme. Pour the mixture over the meat and vegetables. Top everything with a pie crust and slits for vents. Whisk together the egg wash ingredients and brush the mixture at the top of the bowl. Place the pie in the , close the lid, and cook for 1 hour or until the internal temperature reaches 165F. Cover the pie with a foil if it gets too much dark. Let rest for 10 minutes before serving.

Nutrition Info: Calories 371, Total fat 20g, Saturated fat 8g, Total carbs 33g, Net carbs 29g Protein 16g, Sugars 5g, Fiber 4g, Sodium 671mg

429. Pork Carnitas

Servings: 6   Cooking Time: 3 Hours
Ingredients:
- Lime wedges
- 3 jalapeno pepper, minced
- A handful of cilantro, chopped
- 1 cup of chicken broth
- 2 Tbsp olive oil
- Corn tortilla
- 3lb pork shoulder, cut into cubes
- Queso Fresco, crumbled
- 2 Tbsp pork rubs

Directions:
Preheat wood pellet smoker-grill to 300°F. Mop the rub over the pork shoulder. Place pork shoulder in a cast-iron Dutch oven and pour in chicken broth. Transfer pot to grill grate and cook 2½ hours, until fork tender. Remove the cover, bring to a boil then reduce the liquid in pot by half. All this happens within 15 minutes. Place a tablespoon of bacon fat on the skillet and fry the pork for about 10 minutes, until crisp. Take out pork and serve with cilantro, jalapeno, lime, queso fresco, and corn tortillas.

Nutrition Info: Per Serving: Calories: 254kcal, Carbs: 6g, Fat: 6g, Protein: 41g

430. Chipotle Honey Smoked Beef Roast

Servings: 10   Cooking Time: 4 Hours And 20 Minutes
Ingredients:
- Beef roast (5-lbs., 2.3-kg.)
- The Rub Vegetable oil – 2 tablespoons
- Black pepper – 1½ tablespoons
- Salt – 1½ tablespoons
- Brown sugar – ¾ tablespoon
- Onion powder – ¾ tablespoon
- Mustard – 1 teaspoon
- Garlic powder – 1½ teaspoons
- Chipotle powder – 1½ teaspoons
- The Glaze Honey – ½ cup
- Water – 2 tablespoons
- Minced garlic – 1½ tablespoons

Directions:
Place the rub ingredients—vegetable oil, black pepper, salt, brown sugar, onion powder, mustard, garlic powder, and chipotle powder in a bowl then mix until combined. Rub the beef roast with the spice mixture then set aside. Plug the wood pellet smoker and place wood pellet inside the hopper. Turn the switch on. Set the "Smoke" setting and prepare the wood pellet smoker for indirect heat. Wait until the smoke is ready and adjust the temperature to 275°F (135°C). Once the wood pellet smoker has reached the desired temperature, place the seasoned beef roast directly on the grate inside the wood pellet smoker and smoke for 2 hours. In the meantime, combine honey, water, and minced garlic in a bowl then stir until incorporated. After 2 hours, take the beef roast out of the wood pellet smoker and place on as sheet of aluminum foil. Leave the wood pellet smoker on and adjust the temperature to 300°F (149°C). Baste the beef roast with the glaze mixture then wrap it with the aluminum foil. Return the wrapped beef roast to the wood pellet smoker then smoke for another 2 hours. Once the internal temperature of the smoked beef roast has reached 165°F (74°C), remove it from the wood pellet smoker. Let the smoked beef roast rest for about 10 minutes then unwrap it. Transfer the smoked beef roast to a serving dish then serve. Enjoy!

Nutrition Info: Calories: 90 Cal Fat: 3 g Carbohydrates: 1 g   Protein: 14 g Fiber: 0 g

431. Pork Fennel Burger

Servings: 4   Cooking Time: 30 Minutes
Ingredients:
- 1 fennel bulb, trimmed and cut into large chunks
- 3 to 4 garlic cloves
- 2½ pounds boneless pork shoulder, with some of the fat, cut into 1-inch cubes
- 1 tablespoon fennel seeds
- 1 teaspoon caraway seeds (optional)
- 1 teaspoon salt
- ½ teaspoon pepper, or more to taste
- Peeled orange slices to garnish (optional)
- Chopped olives to garnish (optional)
- Chopped parsley to garnish (optional)
- Chopped roasted red pepper to garnish (optional)
- Fennel slices, to garnish (optional)

Directions:
Put fennel and garlic into a food processor and pulse until just chopped; remove to a large bowl. Put pork fat in processor and grind until just chopped; add to bowl. Working in batches, process meat with fennel seeds, caraway, if using and salt and pepper, until meat is just chopped (be careful not to over-process). Add to bowl and mix well. Shape mixture into 8 patties. Supply your smoker with wood pellets and follow the manufacturer's specific start-up procedure. Preheat, with the lid closed, to 425°FArrange the burgers directly on one side of the grill, close the lid, and smoke for 10 minutes. Flip and smoke with the lid closed for 10 to 15

minutes more, or until a meat thermometer inserted in the burgers reads 160°F. Add another Gruyère slice to the burgers during the last 5 minutes of smoking to melt. Garnish with peeled orange slices, chopped olives, chopped parsley, chopped roasted red pepper and fennel slices, to taste.

432. Texas-style Brisket Rub

Servings: 1   Cooking Time: 15 Minutes
Ingredients:
- 2 tsp Sugar
- 2 Tbsp Kosher salt
- 2 tsp Chilli powder
- 2 Tbsp Black pepper
- Tbsp Cayenne pepper
- Tbsp Powdered garlic
- tsp Grounded cumin
- 2 Tbsp Powdered onion
- 1/4 cup paprika, smoked

Directions:
Mix all the ingredients in a small bowl until it is well blended.   Transfer to an airtight jar or container. Store in a cool place.
Nutrition Info: Per Serving: Calories: 18kcal, Carbs: 2g, Fat: 1g, Protein: 0.6g

433. Green Smoothie

Servings: 3 To 4   Cooking Time: 5 Minutes
Ingredients:
- 1/4 cup Baby Spinach
- 1/2 cup Ice
- 1/4 cup Kale
- 1/2 cup Pineapple Chunks
- 1/2 cup Coconut Water
- 1/2 cup mango, diced
- 1/2 banana, diced

Directions:
Begin by placing all the ingredients needed to make the smoothie in the blender pitcher.   Now, press the 'extract' button.   Transfer the smoothie into the serving glass.
Nutrition Info: Calories: 184 Fat: 1.3 g Total Carbs: 44.6 g Fiber: 4.5 g Sugar: 21.9 g Protein: 4.3 g Cholesterol: 0

434. Sweetbread Skewers With Lemon

Servings: 8   Cooking Time: 1 Hour 30 Minutes
Ingredients:
- 1½ pounds veal or lamb sweetbreads
- 1tablespoon salt
- 1tablespoon black peppercorns
- 2lemons, 1 halved and 1 cut into small wedges
- 2tablespoons good-quality olive oil

Directions:
Put the sweetbreads in a large bowl and cover with cold water. Soak in the refrigerator for at least 2 hours or overnight, changing the water several times to remove any blood. Drain and rinse.   Prepare an ice bath in a large bowl. In a large pot, combine 8 cups water, the salt, and the peppercorns. Squeeze the juice from the lemon halves into the water and add the reamed-out shells as well. Bring to a boil, reduce the heat to a very gentle simmer (bubbles just barely breaking the surface), and add the sweetbreads. Poach just until firm, 6 to 10 minutes. Drain and transfer to the ice water to stop the cooking.   When the sweetbreads have cooled, using your fingers, pull away as much of the membrane as you can, along with any fat, gristle, and hard bits. Break the sweetbreads into 1- to 2-inch pieces. (They will largely come apart on their own.) Toss with the oil. (You can prepare them to this point up to a day before cooking; cover and refrigerate.)   If you're using bamboo or wooden skewers, soak them in water for 30 minutes. Meanwhile, start the coals or heat a gas grill for medium direct cooking. Make sure the grates are clean. Alternate 2 or 3 pieces of sweetbreads per skewer, depending on their size, with a wedge of lemon. Put the skewers on the grill directly over the fire. Close the lid and cook, turning several times, until the sweetbreads are crisp on the outside and heated through, 8 to 15 minutes total, depending on the size of the pieces. Serve hot or warm for the best flavor.
Nutrition Info: Calories: 267 Fats: 23 g Cholesterol: 0 mg Carbohydrates: 0 g Fiber: 0 g Sugars: 0 g Proteins: 14 g

435. Smoked Pork Loin In Sweet-beer Marinade

Servings: 6   Cooking Time: 3 Hours
Ingredients:
- Marinade
- 1 onion finely diced
- 1/4 cup honey (preferably a darker honey)
- 1 1/2 cups of dark beer
- 4 Tbs of mustard
- 1 Tbs fresh thyme finely chopped
- Salt and pepper
- Pork 3 1/2 pounds of pork loin

Directions:
Combine all ingredients for the marinade in a bowl.   Place the pork along with marinade mixture in a container and refrigerate overnight. Remove the pork from marinade and dry on kitchen towel.   Prepare the grill on Smoke with the lid open until the fire is established (4 to 5 minutes).   The temperature must reach 250 degrees Fahrenheit and preheat, lid closed, for 10 to 15 minutes.   Place the pork on the grill rack and smoke until the internal temperature of the pork is at least 145-150 ℉ (medium-rare), 2-1/2 to 3 hours.   Remove meat from the smoker and let rest for 15 minutes before slicing.   Serve hot or cold.
Nutrition Info: Calories: 444.6 Cal Fat: 12.7 g Carbohydrates: 17 g   Protein: 60.5 g Fiber: 0.8 g

436. Reverse-seared Tilapia

Servings: 4   Cooking Time: 20 Minutes
Ingredients:
- tilapia fillets
- 2 Tbsp melted butter (unsalted)
- 1/2 cup of all-purpose flour
- Salt and pepper to taste

Directions:
Preheat the wood pellet smoker-grill for direct cooking at 350 F using any pellet   Rinse the fillets and pat dry with a paper towel. Season with salt and pepper, coat with the flour.   Transfer Tilapia fillets to cooking grate and grill for 20 minutes or until internal temperature measure 150 F. Then set fillets aside and increase the temperature of the grill to 450 F   Sear the tilapia for 4 minutes per side or until it flakes. Brush melted butter on the tilapia.   Serve.
Nutrition Info: Per Serving: Calories: 295kcal, Carbs: 11.2g, Fat: 16g, Protein: 24.6g

437. Grilled Pineapple With Chocolate Sauce

Servings: 6 To 8   Cooking Time: 25 Minutes
Ingredients:
- 1pineapple
- 8 oz bittersweet chocolate chips
- 1/2 cup spiced rum
- 1/2 cup whipping cream
- 2tbsp light brown sugar

Directions:
Preheat pellet grill to 400°F.   De-skin the pineapple and slice pineapple into 1 in cubes.   In a saucepan, combine chocolate chips. When chips begin to melt, add rum to the saucepan. Continue to stir until combined, then add a splash of the pineapple's juice.   Add in whipping cream and continue to stir the mixture. Once the sauce is smooth and thickening, lower heat to simmer to keep warm.   Thread pineapple cubes onto skewers. Sprinkle skewers with brown sugar.   Place skewers on the grill grate. Grill for about 5 minutes per side, or until grill marks begin to develop.   Remove skewers from grill and allow to rest on a plate for about 5 minutes. Serve alongside warm chocolate sauce for dipping.
Nutrition Info: Calories: 112.6 Fat: 0.5 g Cholesterol: 0 Carbohydrate: 28.8 g Fiber: 1.6 g Sugar: 0.1 g Protein: 0.4 g

438. Worcestershire Mop And Spritz

Servings: 1 Cup   Cooking Time: 5 Minutes
Ingredients:
- ½ cup water
- ½ cup Worcestershire sauce
- 2 garlic cloves, sliced

Directions:
In a small bowl, stir together the water, Worcestershire sauce, and garlic until mixed.   Transfer to a spray bottle for spritzing. Refrigerate any unused spritz for up to 3 days and use for all kinds of meats.

439. Smoked Pork Shoulder

Servings: 8   Cooking Time: 7 Hours
Ingredients:
- 2 tsp of garlic powder
- 4 tsp of salt, either sea and kosher
- 2 tsp of onion powder
- 4 tsp of black pepper
- 2 tsp of garlic
- 6 pounds of pork shoulder
- 1 tsp of cayenne pepper
- Carolina vinegar sauce
- 11 sesame seed buns, already split
- 3 Tbsp of melted butter.

Directions:
Preheat the grill for 15 minutes at 245°F. Use apple wood pellets for a distinctive, strong woody taste.   Mix onion powder, pepper, garlic powder, cayenne, salt, and black pepper in a bowl. Use your fingers to rub the mixture on the meat.   Place the pork shoulder inside the grill and smoke for 7 hours.   Slice the pork, and the bones will remove effortlessly.   Put the shredded pork in a plate, add sauce and stir it together   Serve it with butter and toasted buns.
Nutrition Info: Per Serving: Calories: 203kcal, Fat: 25g, Carbs: 30g, Protein: 16g

440. Apple Crisp

Servings: 15   Cooking Time: 1 Hour
Ingredients:
- Apple
- 10 apples, washed, peeled and cored
- 1/2 cup four
- 1 cup dark brown sugar
- 1/2 tbsp cinnamon
- 1/2 cup butter
- Crisp
- 3 cups oatmeal, old fashioned
- 1-1/2 cups flour
- 1-1/2 cups salted butter
- 1-1/2 tbsp cinnamon
- Cups brown sugar

Directions:
Preheat your   to 350F.   Slice the apples into cubes then toss with flour, sugar, and cinnamon   Spray cooking spray on a 10x12 foil grill pan, then place the apples in it.place the butter randomly on the apples. In a mixing bowl, mix the crisp ingredients until well combined. Place the mixture over the apples.   Place the grill pan at the hottest part of the   and cook while checking every 20 minutes.   Remove the pan from the when the edges are bubbly, the topping is golden brown and the apples are tender.   Let rest for 25 minutes before serving.

Nutrition Info: Calories 528, Total fat 26g, Saturated fat 16g, Total carbs 75g, Net carbs 70g Protein 4g, Sugars 51g, Fiber 5g, Sodium 209mg

441. Salt-seared Kobe Beef With Tarragon Shallot Butter

Servings: 4   Cooking Time: 40 Minutes
Ingredients:
- 1 (8-inch) square salt block
- 3 Tbsp Unsalted butter
- 2 finely chopped shallot
- 12 oz. Kobe beef, boneless, trimmed, then boiled
- Grounded black pepper to taste
- 1/4 cup of dry vermouth
- Finely chopped tarragon leaves (1 sprig)

Directions:
Preheat the wood pellet smoker-grill for direct cooking at 400 F using any pellet   Heat the salt block on the smoker-grill for 10 minutes, increase the temperature to 450 F (High), and heat for another 10 minutes. While the salt is heating, transfer your beef to a freezer for 10-15 minutes. Do not allow to freeze.   Place a medium skillet on the cooking grate, then add the vermouth and shallot. Stir occasionally to prevent the shallot from boiling dry. Boil until 1 tbsp of shallot remains in the skillet, stir in the pepper and tarragon. Allow to cool and mix with butter.   Remove the beef and slice to about 1/4 -inch-thickness. Sear for 5 minutes per side on the salt block. Serve with shallot-tarragon butter.

Nutrition Info: Per Serving: Calories: 342kcal, Carbs: 16g, Fat: 12g, Protein: 32g

442. Pan-seared Lamb Loins With Horseradish Potato Gratin

Servings: 6   Cooking Time: 2hours
Ingredients:
- 2 lamb loins
- 2 Tbsp Olive oil
- 1-1/2 Tbsp Pepper
- 1-1/2 Tbsp Salt.
- 2 Tbsp prepared horseradish
- Tbsp Unsalted butter
- 1/2 cup of crumbled goat cheese
- 1 cup of whipped cream
- potatoes, peeled and sliced
- 1/2 cup of parmesan cheese

Directions:
Preheat the wood pellet smoker-grill for direct cooking at 300 F using any pellet.   Rinse the lamb chops and pat dry with a paper towel, season with salt and pepper. Grill the lamb loins for 15 minutes, then set the temperature of the grill to High   Place an iron skillet on the cooking grid, add olive oil, then sear the lamb for 10 minutes until brown on all sides. Perform this action carefully to prevent the lamb from burning; it will develop a bitter taste.   Allow it to rest before slicing. Grease a large baking dish with butter. In a large bowl,

combine the cream, parmesan cheese, goat cheese, horseradish, salt, and pepper. Whisk together and drop the sliced potatoes into the mixture.   Arrange the potatoes in the baking dish and cover with plastic wrap, then add a layer of aluminum foil and bake for 1 hour. Remove the cover and bake for another 30 minutes. Serve with the lamb.

Nutrition Info: Per Serving: Calories: 467kcal, Carbs: 28.9g, Fat: 25g, Protein: 42.6g

443. Fall Season Apple Pie

Servings: 8   Cooking Time: 1 Hour
Ingredients:
- 8 C. apples, peeled, cored and sliced thinly
- ¾ C. sugar
- 1 tbsp. fresh lemon juice
- 1 tsp. ground cinnamon
- ¼ tsp. ground nutmeg
- 2 whole frozen pie crusts, thawed
- ¼ C. apple jelly
- 2 tbsp. apple juice
- 2 tbsp. heavy whipping cream

Directions:
Set the temperature of Grill to 375 degrees F and preheat with closed lid for 15 minutes.   In a bowl, add the apples, sugar, lemon juice, flour, cinnamon, and nutmeg and mix well.   Roll the pie crust dough into two (11-inch) circles.   Arrange 1 dough circle into a 9-inch pie plate.   Spread the apple jelly over dough evenly and top with apple mixture.   Dampen the edges of dough crust with apple juice.   Cover with the top crust, pressing the edges together to seal.   Trim the pastry, and flute the edges.   With a sparing knife, make several small slits in the top crust.   Brush the top of the pie with the cream.   Place the pie pan onto the grill and cook for about 50-60 minutes.   Remove from the grill and place the pie onto a wire rack to cool slightly. Serve warm.

Nutrition Info: Calories per serving: 419; Carbohydrates: 79.5g; Protein: 2.2g; Fat: 12.3g; Sugar: 54.2g; Sodium: 214mg; Fiber: 6.1g

444. Ginger And Chili Grilled Shrimp

Servings: 6   Cooking Time: 1 Hour 15 Minutes
Ingredients:
- 1 tsp of salt, kosher
- 2 mangos, riped, peeled, and chopped
- 1 Tbsp of fresh ginger, grated
- 2 cloves of garlic, crushed
- 1-1/4 pound of jumbo shrimp, deveined and peeled.
- 2 jalapenos, chopped
- 1/2 cup of buttermilk, low-fat
- 1/2 tsp of black pepper, ground
- 1 lime, small and also cut into wedges (6)

Directions:
Set the grill for direct cooking at 150°F. Use hickory wood pellets for a robust taste.   Pour the ginger into a bowl,

add buttermilk, jalapenos, garlic, pepper, and salt. Mix thoroughly. Put shrimps inside the same bowl, and mix well with a wooden spoon. Allow it to marinate in the refrigerator for an hour   Arrange 2 mango chops, 3 shrimps on a water-soaked wooden skewer. Do this for the other 5 skewers.   Place shrimp skewers on the grates and grill for 10 minutes, or until the shrimps turn opaque. Serve immediately with the lime wedge

Nutrition Info: Per Serving: Calories: 80kcal, Protein: 20g, Fat:1.3g, Carb: 1.2g

445. Smoked Tuna

Servings: 6   Cooking Time: 3 Hours
Ingredients:
- 2 cups water
- 1 cup brown sugar
- 1 cup salt
- 1 tablespoon lemon zest
- 6 tuna fillets

Directions:
Mix water, brown sugar, salt and lemon zest in a bowl. Coat the tuna fillets with the mixture.   Refrigerate for 6 hours.   Rinse the tuna and pat dry with paper towels. Preheat the   wood pellet grill to 180 degrees F for 15 minutes while the lid is closed.   Smoke the tuna for 3 hours.   Tips: You can also soak tuna in the brine for 24 hours.

446. Lemon Butter Mop For Seafood

Servings: 1 And 1/2 Cups   Cooking Time: 5 Minutes
Ingredients:
- 8 tablespoons (1 stick) butter
- Juice of 1 small lemon
- 1 tablespoon fine salt
- 1½ teaspoons garlic powder
- 1½ teaspoons dried dill weed

Directions:
In a small skillet over medium heat, melt the butter. Stir in the lemon juice, salt, garlic powder, and dill, stirring until well mixed. Use immediately.

447. Grilled Scallion Salad

Servings: 4-6   Cooking Time: 20 Minutes
Ingredients:
- 1/3 cup of rice vinegar
- 2 tsp of sugar
- 1 Tbsp of sesame oil
- 1 Tbsp of gochugaru
- 1 pound of scallion, untrimmed
- 1 Tbsp of sesame seeds

Directions:
Set the grill for indirect cooking at 250°F. Use hickory wood pellets to give scallions a robust taste.   Brush sesame oil on scallions, then arrange it on the cooking grid. Grill with for about 8 minutes.   Remove scallions

from heat and rub with sugar, vinegar, sesame seeds, and vinegar. Serve immediately.

Nutrition Info: Per Serving: Calories: 56kcal, Carbs: 13g, Fat: 7g, Protein: -g

448. Berry Cobbler On A Pellet Grill

Servings: 8   Cooking Time: 35 Minutes
Ingredients:
- For fruit filling
- 3cups frozen mixed berries
- 1lemon juice
- 1cup brown sugar
- 1tbsp vanilla extract
- 1bsp lemon zest, finely grated
- Apinch of salt
- Forcobbler topping
- 1-1/2 cups all-purpose flour
- 1-1/2 tbsp baking powder
- 3tbsp sugar, granulated
- 1/2 tbsp salt
- 8tbsp cold butter
- 1/2 cup sour cream
- 2tbsp raw sugar

Directions:
Set your pellet grill on "smoke" for about 4-5 minutes with the lid open until fire establishes, and your grill starts smoking.   Preheat your grill to 350 F for about 10-15 minutes with the grill lid closed.   Meanwhile, combine frozen mixed berries, Lemon juice, brown sugar, vanilla, lemon zest, and a pinch of salt.   Transfer into a skillet and let the fruit sit and thaw.   Mix flour, baking powder, sugar, and salt in a bowl, medium. Cut cold butter into peas sizes using a pastry blender then add to the mixture. Stir to mix everything together.   Stir in sour cream until dough starts coming together.   Pinch small pieces of dough and place over the fruit until fully covered. Splash the top with raw sugar.   Now place the skillet directly on the grill grate, close the lid and cook for about 35 minutes until juices bubble, and a golden-brown dough topping.   Remove the skillet from the pellet grill and cool for several minutes.   Scoop and serve warm.

Nutrition Info: Calories: 371 Total Fat: 13g Saturated Fat: 8g Total Carbs: 60g Net Carbs: 58g Protein: 3g Sugars: 39g Fiber: 2g Sodium: 269mg

449. Pork Dry Rub

Servings: 1   Cooking Time: 15 Minutes
Ingredients:
- Tbsp Kosher salt
- 2 Tbsp Powered onions
- Tbsp Cayenne pepper
- 1tsp Dried mustard
- 1/4 cup brown sugar
- Tbsp Powdered garlic
- Tbsp Powdered chili pepper
- 1/4 cup smoked paprika
- 2 Tbsp Black pepper

Directions:
Combine all the ingredients in a small bowl.   Transfer to an airtight jar or container.   Keep stored in a cool, dry place.
Nutrition Info: Per Serving: Calories: 16kcal, Carbs: 3g, Fat:0.9g, Protein: 0.8g

450. Super-addicting Mushrooms

Servings: 4   Cooking Time: 45 Minutes
Ingredients:
- 4 C. fresh whole baby Portobello mushrooms, cleaned
- 1 tbsp. canola oil
- 1 tsp. granulated garlic
- 1 tsp. onion powder
- Salt and freshly ground black pepper, to taste

Directions:
Set the temperature of   Grill to 180 degrees F and preheat with closed lid for 15 minutes, using charcoal. In a bowl, add all ingredients and mix well.   Place the mushrooms onto the grill and cook for about 30 minutes. Remove the mushrooms from grill.   Now, preheat the Grill to 400 degrees F and preheat with closed lid for 15 minutes.   Place the mushrooms onto the grill and cook for about 15 minutes.   Remove the mushrooms from grill and serve warm.
Nutrition Info: Calories per serving: 50; Carbohydrates: 3.3g; Protein: 2.4g; Fat: 3.7g; Sugar: 1.6g; Sodium: 43mg; Fiber: 0.8g

451. Smoked Mac And Cheese

Servings: 8   Cooking Time: 1 Hour
Ingredients:
- 1/2 cup butter, salted
- 1/3 cup flour
- 1/2 tbsp salt
- 6 cups whole milk
- Dash of Worcestershire
- 1/2 tbsp dry mustard
- 1 lb small cooked shells, al dente in well-salted water
- 2 cups white cheddar, smoked
- 2 cups cheddar jack cheese
- 1 cup crushed ritz

Directions:
Set your grill on "smoke" and run for about 5-10 minutes with the lid open until fire establishes. Now turn your grill to 325 F then close the lid.   Melt butter in a saucepan, medium, over low--medium heat then whisk in flour.   Cook while whisking for about 5-6 minutes over low heat until light tan color.   Whisk in salt, milk, Worcestershire, and mustard over low-medium heat stirring frequently until a thickened sauce.   Stir noodles, small shells, white sauce, and 1 cup cheddar cheese in a large baking dish, 10x3" high-sided, coated with butter.   Top with 1 cup cheddar cheese and ritz. Place on the grill and bake for about 25-30 minutes until

a bubbly mixture and cheese melts.   Serve immediately. Enjoy!
Nutrition Info: Calories 628, Total fat 42g, Saturated fat 24g, Total carbs 38g, Net carbs 37g, Protein 25g, Sugars 11g, Fiber 1g, Sodium 807mg, Potassium 699mg

452. Smoked Pork Ribs With Fresh Herbs

Servings: 6   Cooking Time: 3 Hours
Ingredients:
- 1/4 cup olive oil
- 1 Tbs garlic minced
- 1 Tbs crushed fennel seeds
- 1 tsp of fresh basil leaves finely chopped
- 1 tsp fresh parsley finely chopped
- 1 tsp fresh rosemary finely chopped
- 1 tsp fresh sage finely chopped
- Salt and ground black pepper to taste
- 3 pounds pork rib roast bone-in

Directions:
Combine spices and mix well   Coat chop with mixture Start the pellet grill Set temperature to 225 ℉ and preheat, lid closed, for 10 to 15 minutes.   Smoke the ribs for 3 hours.   Place the ribs to you preferred container and serve while it is hot
Nutrition Info: Calories: 459.2 Cal Fat: 31.3 g Carbohydrates: 0.6 g   Protein: 41 g Fiber: 0.03 g

453. Smoked Beef Stew

Servings: 6-8   Cooking Time: 4 Hours
Ingredients:
- 2 ½ lbs. Beef Roast, sliced into 1 -inch cubes
- 2 Potatoes for boiling, cut into pieces (peeled)
- 4 Carrots cut into pieces (peeled)
- 1 ½ tsp. Thyme, dried
- 1 - 2 Bay leaves
- 2 tsp. of Worcestershire sauce
- 1 tbsp. of Tomato paste
- 2 Garlic cloves, minced
- 1 onion sliced lengthwise
- 3 cups Beef broth, low sodium
- Optional: ½ cup of Red wine
- 2 tbsp. Oil
- Black pepper and salt
- 2 tbsp. of Flour
- 2 - 3 tbsp. Potato flakes
- For serving: Buttered noodles or Biscuits
- For Garnish: Parsley, chopped

Directions:
In a bag add the flour, salt, and black pepper to taste. Add the meat pieces. Toss and coat.   Heat the oil in a large pot until hot. Add the meat pieces. Cook until browned. Add the wine, broth and scrape the brown bits using a wooden spoon. Add thyme, bay leaves, Worcestershire, tomato paste, garlic, and onion. Cover the pot.   Preheat the grill to 300F with the lid closed.   Put pot on grate and cook 2 hours. After 2 hours add the potatoes and carrots. Cook until the veggies and meat are tender, 2 hours more.   If you

need to thicken the gravy add 2 - 3 tbsp. Potato flakes.   Serve garnished with parsley.
Nutrition Info: Calories: 240 Cal Fat: 11 g Carbohydrates: 17 g   Protein: 19 g Fiber: 3 g

454. Smoked Sriracha Sauce

Servings: 2   Cooking Time: 1 Hour
Ingredients:
- 1 lb Fresno chiles, stems pulled off and seeds removed
- 1/2 cup rice vinegar
- 1/2 cup red wine vinegar
- 1 carrot, medium and cut into rounds, 1/4 inch
- 1-1/2 tbsp sugar, dark-brown
- 4 garlic cloves, peeled
- 1 tbsp olive oil
- 1 tbsp kosher salt
- 1/2 cup water

Directions:
Smoke chiles in a smoker for about 15 minutes.   Bring to boil both vinegars then add carrots, sugar, and garlic. Simmer for about 15 minutes while covered. Cool for 30 minutes.   Place the chiles, olive oil, vinegar-vegetable mixture, salt, and 1/4 cup water into a blender.   Blend for about 1-2 minutes on high. Add remaining water and blend again. You can add another 1/4 cup water if you want your sauce thinner.   Pour the sauce into jars and place in a refrigerator.   Serve.
Nutrition Info: Calories 147, Total fat 5.23g, Saturated fat 0.7g, Total carbs 21g, Net carbs 18g, Protein 3g, Sugar 13g, Fiber 3g, Sodium: 671mg

455. Native Southern Cornbread

Servings: 8   Cooking Time: 20 Minutes
Ingredients:
- 2 tbsp. butter
- 1½ C. all-purpose flour
- 1½ C. yellow cornmeal
- 2 tbsp. sugar
- 3 tsp. baking powder
- ¾ tsp. baking soda
- ¾ tsp. salt
- 1 C. whole milk
- 1 C. buttermilk
- 3 large eggs
- 3 tbsp. butter, melted

Directions:
Set the temperature of   Grill to 400 degrees F and preheat with closed lid for 15 minutes.   In a 13x9-inch baking dish, place 2 tbsp. of butter.   Place the baking dish onto grill to melt butter and heat up the pan.   In a large bowl, mix together flour, cornmeal, sugar, baking powder, baking soda and salt.   In another bowl, add milk, buttermilk, eggs and melted butter and beat until well combined.   Add the egg mixture into flour mixture and mix until just moistened.   Carefully, remove the heated baking dish from grill.   Place the bread mixture into heated baking dish evenly.   Place

the pan onto the grill and cook for about 20 minutes or until a toothpick inserted in the center comes out clean. Remove from grill and place the pan onto a wire rack to cool for about 10 minutes.   Carefully, invert the bread onto the wire rack to cool completely before slicing. Cut the bread into desired-sized slices and sere.
Nutrition Info: Calories per serving: 302; Carbohydrates: 42.4g; Protein: 8.7g; Fat: 10.4g; Sugar: 6.4g; Sodium: 467mg; Fiber: 2.3g

456. Smoked Chicken With Perfect Poultry Rub

Servings: 2   Cooking Time: 3 Hours 15 Minutes
Ingredients:
- 2 Tbsp of onion, powder
- 1/4 cup of black pepper, freshly ground
- 2 Tbsp of dry mustard
- 3/4 cup of paprika
- 4pound chicken
- 3 lemon
- 2 tsp of cayenne
- 1/4 cup of sugar
- 1/4 cup of celery salt

Directions:
In a bowl, mix the onion powder, paprika, black pepper, dry mustard, cayenne, sugar, celery, salt, and 2 lemons. Add your chicken to the rub and slice some parts so that the ingredients will find their way in.   Preheat the grill for 15 minutes at 225°F. Use apple wood pellets for a distinctive, strong woody taste.   Place the coated chicken on the preheated grill and smoke for 3 hours or until internal temperature reads 160°F.   Allow chicken to cool, then serve.
Nutrition Info: Per Serving: Calories: 255kcal, Protein: 35g, Carbs: 42g, Fat: 35g.

457. Empanadas

Servings: 4   Cooking Time: 20 Minutes
Ingredients:
- 3/4 cup + 1 tbsp all-purpose flour
- ½ tsp baking powder
- 1tbsp sugar
- ¼ tsp salt or to taste
- 2tbsp cold water
- 1/3 cups butter
- 1small egg (beaten)
- Filling:
- ½ small onion (chopped)
- 57 g ground beef (1/8 pound)
- 2tbsp marinara sauce
- 1small carrot peeled and diced)
- 1/8 small potato (peeled and diced) 35 grams
- 2tbsp water
- 1garlic clove (minced)
- 1tbsp olive oil
- 1tbsp raisin
- 2tbsp green peas
- ½ tsp salt or taste

- 1/2 tsp ground black pepper or to taste
- 1 hard-boiled egg (sliced)

Directions:
Start your grill on smoke mode and leave the lid open for 5 minutes, or until fire starts.   Close the grill and preheat grill to 400°F with the lid closed for 15 minutes, using hickory hardwood pellets.   For the fillet, place a cast iron skillet on the grill and add the oil.   Once the oil is hot, add the onion and garlic and sauté until the onion is tender and translucent.   Add the ground beef and sauté until it is tender, stirring often.   Stir in the marinara, salt, water, and pepper.   Bring to a boil and reduce the heat. Cook for 30 seconds.   Stir in the carrot, raisin, and potatoes and cook for 3 minutes.   Stir in the green peas and sliced egg. Cook for additional 2 minutes, stirring often.   Spray a baking dish with a non-stick spray.   For the dough, combine the flour, baking powder salt and sugar in a large mixing bowl. Mix until well combined.   Add butter and mix until it is well incorporated.   Add egg and mix until you form the dough.   Put the dough on a floured surface and knead the dough for a few minutes. Add more flour if the dough is not thick enough.   Roll the dough flat with a rolling pin. The flat dough should be ¼ inch thick.   Cut the flat dough into circles.   Add equal amounts of the beef mixture to the middle of each flat circular dough slice. Fold the dough slice and close the edges by pressing with your fingers or a fork.   Arrange the empanadas into the baking sheet in a single layer.   Place the baking sheet on the grill and bake for 10 minutes.   Remove the baking sheet from the grill and flip the empanadas. Bake for another 10 minutes on the grill or until empanadas are golden brown.

Nutrition Info: Calories: 353 Total Fat: 22.3 g Saturated Fat: 11.3 g Cholesterol: 129 mg Sodium: 481 mg Total Carbohydrate 28.9 g Dietary Fiber 1.9 g Total Sugars: 6.6 g Protein: 10.4 g

458. Texas Styled Smoked Flounder

Servings: 6   Cooking Time: 20 Minutes
Ingredients:
- 1 whole flounder
- 1 halved lemon
- Ground black pepper as needed
- 2 tablespoons of chopped up fresh dill
- 1 tablespoon of olive oil
- 1 cup of soaked wood chips

Directions:
Preheat your smoker to a temperature of 350 degrees Fahrenheit.   Slice half of your lemon and place them into the slices. Rub the fish with a coating of olive oil. Squeeze another half of the lemon all over the fish. Season with some black pepper.   Rub 1 tablespoon of dill into the slits and insert the lemon slices firmly. Place the flounder on top of a large piece of aluminum foil and fold the sides all around the fish.   Place the fish in your smoker and throw a couple handful of soaked wood chips into the coals. And smoke for 10 minutes   Once done, seal up the foil and smoke it until it is fully done. Remove fish and garnish with some extra dill

Nutrition Info: Calories: 226 Cal Fat: 4 g Carbohydrates: 28 g   Protein: 28 g Fiber: 0 g

459. Smoked Ribs

Servings: 8   Cooking Time: 6 Hours
Ingredients:
- 4 baby back ribs
- 1 cup pork rub
- 1 cup barbecue sauce

Directions:
Preheat your grill to 180 degrees F for 15 minutes while the lid is closed.   Sprinkle baby back ribs with pork rub. Smoke the ribs for 5 hours.   Brush the ribs with barbecue sauce.   Wrap the ribs with foil.   Put the ribs back to the grill.   Increase temperature to 350 degrees F.   Cook for 45 minutes to 1 hour.   Let rest before slicing and serving.   Tips: Trim excess fat from the baby back ribs before cooking.

460. Grilled Clam With Lemon-cayenne Butter

Servings: 2   Cooking Time: 15 Minutes
Ingredients:
- 2 tsp of lemon juice, preferably fresh
- Large pinch of salt (kosher)
- 2 dozen of littleneck clams
- 1 large clove of garlic
- Chives, freshly chopped
- 4 Tbsp of unsalted butter, already melted
- Pinch of cayenne pepper

Directions:
Set the grill for direct cooking at 300°F. Use alder wood pellets for mild taste and aroma.   Mash garlic and salt with a mortar and pestle to form a paste.   Scoop the paste into a small bowl and add cayenne pepper, butter, and lemon.   Grill clam over the preheated cooking grid for 5 minutes. When clam is ready, it will open. Carefully transfer opened clam to the bowl containing lemon-cayenne butter. Do not spill the clam-juice when transporting.   Gently mix the clam and butter until it is well-combined.   Serve immediately with chives.

Nutrition Info: Per Serving: Calories: 148kcal, Carbs: 31g, Fat: 19g, Protein: 25g

461. Honey Cured Ham Ribs

Servings: 3   Cooking Time: 5 Hours 20 Minutes
Ingredients:
- 3/4 cup of honey
- 1-1/2 cup of cold water
- 1-1/2 cup of hot water
- 8 cloves
- 1 rack of spareribs
- 3/4 cup of kosher or sea salt
- 1-1/2 tsp of pink curing salt
- 3 bay leaves
- Mustard seed caviar

Directions:
Place the ribs on the baking sheet. Mix the hot water, honey, coarse salt, and pink curing salt until the salt and honey dissolve in the water. Allow it to cool to room temperature. Add the rib to the cooled brine and transfer it to a Ziploc bag. Keep in the refrigerator for 3 days. Remove the ribs from the refrigerator and place it on the baking pan. Preheat the grill for 15 minutes at 250°F. Use pecan wood pellets for a spicy, nutty taste. Put the ribs on the grates of the grid and smoke for about 4 hours. Serve immediately with mustard seed caviar.
Nutrition Info: Per Serving: Calories: 375kcal, Protein: 45g, Fat: 43.5g, Carbs: 55g

462. Smoked Cheese Dip

Servings: 8   Cooking Time: 1 Hour And 15 Minutes
Ingredients:
- Ice cubes
- 1 block cheddar cheese
- 8 tablespoons butter
- ½ cup carrots, chopped
- 1 onion, chopped
- 1 cup heavy cream
- 3/4 cup flour
- Hot sauce
- 1 teaspoon Worcestershire sauce

Directions:
Preheat your wood pellet grill to 180 degrees F for 15 minutes while the lid is closed. Add ice cubes to a pan. Place a cooling rack on top. Put the cheese block on the rack. Put this on top of the grill. Smoke for 30 minutes. Transfer the cheese to your freezer. In a pan over medium heat, add the butter and let it melt. Cook the onion and carrots for 15 minutes. Stir in the rest of the ingredients. Reduce heat and simmer for 15 minutes. Take the cheese out of the freezer and shred. Put the shredded cheese into the mixture. Stir while cooking until cheese has melted.
Nutrition Info: Calories: 1230 Fats: 77 g Cholesterol: 145 mg Carbohydrates: 104 g Fiber: 8 g Sugar: 7g Protein: 40 g

463. Smoked Pork Cutlets In Citrus-herb Marinade

Servings: 4   Cooking Time: 1 Hour And 45 Minutes
Ingredients:
- 4 pork cutlets
- 1 fresh orange juice
- 2 large lemons freshly squeezed
- 10 twigs of coriander chopped
- 2 Tbs of fresh parsley finely chopped
- 3 cloves of garlic minced
- 2 Tbs of olive oil
- Salt and ground black pepper

Directions:
Place the pork cutlets in a large container along with all remaining ingredients; toss to cover well. Refrigerate at least 4 hours, or overnight. When ready, remove the pork cutlets from marinade and pat dry on kitchen towel. Start pellet grill on, lid open, until the fire is established (4-5 minutes). The temperature must rise up to 250 degrees Fahrenheit and preheat until 15 minutes at most. Place pork cutlets on grill grate and smoke for 1 1/2 hours.
Nutrition Info: Calories: 260 Cal Fat: 12 g Carbohydrates: 5 g   Protein: 32.2 g Fiber: 0.25 g

464. Peach Blueberry Cobbler

Servings: 4   Cooking Time: 1hour15 Minutes
Ingredients:
- 2 cups of peaches, peeled and sliced
- 1 cup of fresh blueberries
- 1 cup of all-purpose flour
- 1 cup of milk
- 1/2 cup of melted butter, salted
- 2 tsp Baking powder
- 1-1/2 cup sugar
- 1/2 tsp salt
- 1/2 tsp vanilla extract

Directions:
Set the wood pellet smoker-grill to indirect cooking at 375F In a bowl, add blueberry, peaches, and ¾ cup sugar. Stir the mixture until the blueberry is coated. Set aside. In another bowl, combine the other ingredients with the remaining sugar and mix well. Be careful not to over stir the mixture. Pour into the baking dish, add the blueberry-peach mixture on top. Do not stir. Transfer baking pan to the grill and cover with steel construction. Bake for 45-60 minutes, remove and allow to rest before serving.
Nutrition Info: Per Serving: Calories: 474kcal, Carbs: 41g, Fat: 25g, Protein: 21g

465. Twice- Baked Potatoes With Smoked Gouda And Grilled Scallions

Servings: 6   Cooking Time: 1hours 15 Minutes
Ingredients:
- 3 large potatoes
- 8 TbspUnsalted butter
- Tbsp Of barbeque rub
- 1-1/2 cup of smoked gouda cheese (grated)
- 1/4 cup of extra-virgin olive oil
- 3/4 cup heavy cream
- Salt and pepper to taste
- 1/4 cup chopped scallions

Directions:
Set the wood pellet smoker-grill to indirect cooking at 400 F Brush the potatoes with olive oil, make incisions with fork and season with salt. Wrap with aluminum foil paper and bake on grill grates for 30 minutes per side. Transfer to a rimmed sheet and allow to cool. Cut the potatoes lengthwise, scoop out the flesh into a bowl. Add butter and 1 cup of cheese. Set aside. Place a small pot over low-medium heat, add cream, then heat for 1 minute. Add the scallions and the

barbeque rub and mix well   Add the scallion mixture to the potatoes and cheese in the bowl, combine until it is evenly mixed. Scoop the mixture back into the potato shell and top with cheese.   Bake for 5 minutes or until the cheese melts.
Nutrition Info: Per Serving: Calories: 276kcal, Carbs: 28g, Fat: 14.5g, Protein: 3g

466. Smoked Rib Eye With Bourbon Butter

Servings: 4-6   Cooking Time: 1 Hour And 30 Minutes
Ingredients:
- 4 Ribeye steaks (1 inch thick).
- Fresh ground pepper – 1/2 tsp.
- Garlic (minced) – 1-2 cloves.
- Green Onion (finely minced) – 1 tbsp.
- Parsley (finely minced) – 1 tbsp.
- Salt– 1/2 tsp.
- Bourbon – 2 tbsp.
- Butter – 1/2 cup.
- prime rub.

Directions:
In a mixing bowl, add butter, parsley, chives, bourbon, garlic, salt, and pepper. Stir all of the ingredients with a wooden spoon. Put the smoker on.   Until the fire is established, keep the lid open. The fire should be established in about 4-5 minutes.   Season the rib eye steaks with a prime rub. Arrange the steaks on the grill and smoke them for about an hour.   Then temporarily remove the steaks from the smoker and set your smoker's temperature up to 450F. Place the steaks back on the grill. Give one side about 6-8 minutes and then turn it over.   Keep the other side for the same amount of time. Otherwise, if you like your steak medium rare then keep cooking and turning over until the internal temperature is 135 F.   Take the steak out of the smoker after they are cooked to your liking and immediately pat them with the bourbon butter sauce you made earlier.   Let the meat rest for about 3 minutes before serving it.
Nutrition Info: Calories: 230 Cal Fat: 16 g Carbohydrates: 0 g   Protein: 21 g Fiber: 0 g

467. Black Bean Dipping Sauce

Servings: 4   Cooking Time: 10 Minutes
Ingredients:
- 2 tablespoons black bean paste
- 2 tablespoons peanut butter
- 1 tablespoon maple syrup
- 2 tablespoons olive oil

Directions:
In a blender place all ingredients and blend until smooth Pour sauce in a bowl and serve

468. Wood Pellet Spicy Brisket

Servings: 10   Cooking Time: 9 Hours
Ingredients:

- 2 tbsp garlic powder
- 2 tbsp onion powder
- 2 tbsp paprika
- 2 tbsp chili powder
- 1/3 cup salt
- 1/3 cup black pepper
- 12 lb whole packer brisket, trimmed
- 1-1/2 cup beef broth

Directions:
Set your wood pellet temperature to 225°F. Let preheat for 15 minutes with the lid closed.   Meanwhile, mix garlic, onion, paprika, chili, salt, and pepper in a mixing bowl.   the brisket generously on all sides.   Place the meat on the grill with the fat side down and let it cool until the internal temperature reaches 160°F. Remove the meat from the grill and double wrap it with foil. Return it to the grill and cook until the internal temperature reaches 204°F.   Remove from grill, unwrap the brisket and let rest for 15 minutes.   Slice and serve.
Nutrition Info: Calories: 270 Total Fat: 20 g Saturated Fat: 8 g Total Carbs: 3 g Net Carbs: 3 g Protein: 20 g Sugar: 1 g Fiber: 0 g Sodium: 1220mg

469. Mutton Barbecued And Black Dip

Servings: 7   Cooking Time: 7 Hours 20 Minutes
Ingredients:
- Kosher or sea salt
- 7 hamburger buns
- 2 Tbsp of butter
- Sliced dill pickle
- 6 pounds of lamb shoulder
- Black dip

Directions:
Season lamb with salt and pepper   Preheat the grill for 15 minutes at 250°F. Use pecan wood pellets.   Put the lamb inside black dip, then transfer it to the smoking rack. Smoke the lamb for 7 hours.   Put the already smoked lamb on a dish or board. Allow it to rest for 10 minutes. Remove the fat lumps.   Put butter on the buns, pile the lamb on the buns, and add pickle slices. Serve it with black dip.
Nutrition Info: Per Serving: Calories: 279.9kcal, Fat: 30.2g, Protein: 35g, Carbs: 49g

470. Grilled Chili Burger

Servings: 8   Cooking Time: 20 Minutes
Ingredients:
- 1 tsp of chili powder
- 4 tsp of butter
- 2 pounds of round steak, twice-grounded
- 1 clove of garlic
- Salt and ground pepper, preferably freshly ground
- 1/4 cup of bread crumbs

Directions:
Set the grill for direct cooking at 300°F. Use maple pellets for a robust and woody taste.   Pour the meat inside a bowl and add the rest of the ingredients. Mix

until well-combined. Mold the meat mixture to form 8 patties. Arrange patties on the preheated cooking grid and grill for 10 minutes before flipping and grilling the other side for another 10 minutes. Serve immediately with hamburger buns.

Nutrition Info: Per Serving: Calories: 260kcal, Protein: 13g, Fat: 10.5g, Carbs: 29.9g.

471. Rosemary-garlic Lamb Seasoning

Servings: 2   Cooking Time: 5 Minutes
Ingredients:
- 2 teaspoons dried rosemary leaves
- 2 teaspoons coarse kosher salt
- 1 teaspoon garlic powder
- 1 teaspoon freshly ground black pepper
- ½ teaspoon onion powder
- ½ teaspoon dried minced onion

Directions:
In a small airtight container or zip-top bag, combine the rosemary, salt, garlic powder, black pepper, onion powder, and minced onion. Close the container and shake to mix. Unused seasoning will keep in an airtight container for months.

472. Greek Leg Of Lamb

Servings: 12 To 16   Cooking Time: 20 To 25 Minutes
Ingredients:
- 2 tablespoons finely chopped fresh rosemary
- 1 tablespoon ground thyme
- 5 garlic cloves, minced
- 2 tablespoons sea salt
- 1 tablespoon freshly ground black pepper
- Butcher's string
- 1 whole boneless (6- to 8-pound) leg of lamb
- ¼ cup extra-virgin olive oil
- 1 cup red wine vinegar
- ½ cup canola oil

Directions:
In a small bowl, combine the rosemary, thyme, garlic, salt, and pepper; set aside. Using butcher's string, tie the leg of lamb into the shape of a roast. Your butcher should also be happy to truss the leg for you. Rub the lamb generously with the olive oil and season with the spice mixture. Transfer to a plate, cover with plastic wrap, and refrigerate for 4 hours. Remove the lamb from the refrigerator but do not rinse. Supply your smoker with wood pellets and follow the manufacturer's specific start-up procedure. Preheat, with the lid closed, to 325°F. In a small bowl, combine the red wine vinegar and canola oil for basting. Place the lamb directly on the grill, close the lid, and smoke for 20 to 25 minutes per pound (depending on desired doneness), basting with the oil and vinegar mixture every 30 minutes. Lamb is generally served medium-rare to medium, so it will be done when a meat thermometer inserted in the thickest part reads 140°F to 145°F. Let the lamb rest for about 15 minutes before slicing to serve.

473. Smoked Pork Chops Marinated With Tarragon

Servings: 4   Cooking Time: 4-6 Hours
Ingredients:
- 1/2 cup olive oil
- 4 Tbsp of fresh tarragon chopped
- 2 tsp fresh thyme, chopped
- salt and grated black pepper
- 2 tsp apple-cider vinegar
- 4 pork chops or fillets

Directions:
Whisk the olive oil, tarragon, thyme, salt, pepper, apple cider and stir well. Place the pork chops in a container and pour with tarragon mixture. Refrigerate for 2 hours. Start pellet grill on, lid open, until the fire is established (4-5 minutes). The temperature must rise to 250 degrees Fahrenheit with the lid closed until 15 minutes The temperature must rise up to 250 degrees Fahrenheit and must be preheated for at most 15 minutes. Remove chops from marinade and pat dry on kitchen towel. Arrange pork chops on the grill rack and smoke for about 3 to 4 hours. Transfer chops on a serving platter and let rest 15 minutes before serving.

Nutrition Info: Calories: 528.8 Cal Fat: 35 g Carbohydrates: 0.6 g   Protein: 51 g Fiber: 0.14 g

474. Barbecue Bacon Bites

Servings: 4   Cooking Time: 30 Minutes
Ingredients:
- 1 tablespoon ground fennel
- Salt and pepper to taste
- 1/2 cup brown sugar
- 1 lb. pork belly, sliced into cubes

Directions:
Preheat your wood pellet grill to 350 degrees F. for 15 minutes while the lid is closed. In a bowl, mix the ground fennel, salt, pepper and brown sugar. Coat the bacon cubes with this mixture. Grill for 30 minutes. Tips: It's also a good idea to use a foil for cooking the bacon to catch the bacon drippings and reserve for later use.

475. Basil Pesto Sauce

Servings: 4   Cooking Time: 10 Minutes
Ingredients:
- 2 cloves garlic
- 2 oz. basil leaves
- 1 tablespoon pine nuts
- 1 oz. parmesan cheese
- ½ cup olive oil

Directions:
In a blender place all ingredients and blend until smooth Pour sauce in a bowl and serve

476. Grilled Lime Chicken

Servings: 6   Cooking Time: 45 Minutes
Ingredients:
- 2 teaspoon sugar
- 1 teaspoon chili powder
- 1 1/2 teaspoons granulated garlic
- 1 1/2 teaspoons ground cumin
- Salt and pepper to taste
- 12 chicken thighs, skin removed
- 1 1/2 tablespoons olive oil
- 1 1/2 tablespoons butter
- 4 tablespoons pineapple juice
- 4 tablespoons honey
- 1 1/2 tablespoons lime juice
- 1/4 teaspoon red pepper flakes
- 1 1/2 tablespoons hot sauce

Directions:
Set the grill to 375 degrees F. Preheat it for 10 minutes. In a bowl, mix the sugar, chili powder, garlic, cumin, salt and pepper. Coat the chicken with the olive oil and sprinkle with the dry rub. Grill the chicken for 7 minutes per side. In a pan over medium heat, simmer the rest of the ingredients for 10 minutes. Remove from heat and transfer to a bowl. Brush the mixture on both sides of the chicken. Cook for another 7 minutes per side. Tips: Add more hot sauce to the glaze if you want your chicken spicier.

477. Banana Nut Oatmeal

Servings: 2   Cooking Time: 5 Minutes
Ingredients:
- 1/2 tbsp. Maple Syrup
- 1/4 cup Hemp Seeds
- 1/2 cup Steel Cut Oats
- Dash of Sea Salt
- 1 tsp. Vanilla Extract
- 1/2 cup Water
- 1/2 tsp. Cinnamon
- 1 tsp. Nutmeg
- 1/3 cup Milk
- 1 Banana, medium, sliced and divided

Directions:
First, keep half of the banana, salt, oats, vanilla, cinnamon, almond milk, nutmeg, and maple syrup in the blender pitcher. After that, press the 'cook' button and then the 'high' button. Cook for 5 minutes. Once done, divide the oatmeal among the serving bowls and top it with the remaining sliced banana and hempseeds.
Nutrition Info: Fat: 5.3 g Calories: 189 Total Carbs: 34.9 g Fiber: 7.5 g Sugar: 15.3 g Protein: 3.9 g Cholesterol: 0

478. Polish Kielbasa

Servings: 8   Cooking Time: 1 To 2 Hours
Ingredients:
- 4 pounds ground pork
- 1/2 cup water
- 2 garlic cloves, minced
- 4 teaspoons salt
- 1 teaspoon freshly ground black pepper
- 1 teaspoon dried marjoram
- 1/2 teaspoon ground allspice
- 14 feet natural hog casings, medium size

Directions:
In a large bowl, combine the pork, water, garlic, salt, pepper, marjoram, and allspice. Stuff the casings according to the instructions on your sausage stuffing device, or use a funnel (see Tip). Twist the casings according to your desired length and prick each with a pin in several places so the kielbasa won't burst. Transfer the kielbasa to a plate, cover with plastic wrap, and refrigerate for at least 8 hours or overnight. Remove from the refrigerator and allow the links to come to room temperature. Supply your smoker with wood pellets and follow the manufacturer's specific start-up procedure. Preheat, with the lid closed, to 225°F. Place the kielbasa directly on the grill grate, close the lid, and smoke for 1 hour 30 minutes to 2 hours, or until a meat thermometer inserted in each link reads 155°F. (The internal temperature will rise about 5°F when resting, for a finished temp of 160°F.) Serve with buns and condiments of your choosing, or cut up the kielbasa and serve with smoked cabbage

479. Smoked Pork Tenderloin With Mexican Pineapple Sauce

Servings: 6   Cooking Time: 3 Hours And 55 Minutes
Ingredients:
- Pineapple Sauce
- 1 can (11 oz) unsweetened crushed pineapple
- 1 can (11 oz) roasted tomato or tomatillo
- 1/2 cup port wine
- 1/4 cup orange juice
- 1/4 cup packed brown sugar
- 1/4 cup lime juice
- 2 tbsp Worcestershire sauce
- 1 tsp garlic powder
- 1/4 tsp cayenne pepper
- PORK
- 2 pork tenderloin (1 pound each)
- 1 tsp ground cumin
- 1/2 tsp pepper
- 1/4 tsp cayenne pepper
- 2 tbsp lime juice (freshly squeezed)

Directions:
Combine cumin, pepper, cayenne pepper and lime juice and rub over tenderloins. Smoke grill for 4-5 minutes. Preheat, lid closed for 10-15 minutes Smoke tenderloin for 2 ½ to 3 hours. Rest for 5 minutes For Sauce: Combine ingredients and boil for 25 minutes Remove from heat and cool. Serve pork slices with pineapple sauce and lime wedges.
Nutrition Info: Calories: 277.85 Cal Fat: 3.49 g Carbohydrates: 24.31 g Protein: 32.42 g Fiber: 0.67 g

480. Pellet Grill Funeral Potatoes

Servings: 8   Cooking Time: 1 Hour
Ingredients:
- 1, 32 oz, package frozen hash browns
- 1/2 cup cheddar cheese, grated
- 1 can cream of chicken soup
- 1 cup sour cream
- 1 cup Mayonnaise
- 3 cups corn flakes, whole or crushed
- 1/4 cup melted butter

Directions:
Preheat your pellet grill to 350F.   Spray a 13 x 9 baking pan, aluminum, using a cooking spray, non-stick.   Mix together hash browns, cheddar cheese, chicken soup cream, sour cream, and mayonnaise in a bowl, large. Spoon the mixture into a baking pan gently.   Mix corn flakes and melted butter then sprinkle over the casserole. Grill for about 1-1/2 hours until potatoes become tender. If the top browns too much, cover using a foil until potatoes are done.   Remove from the grill and serve hot.

Nutrition Info: Calories: 403 Total Fat: 37 g Saturated Fat: 12 g Total Carbs: 14 g Net Carbs: 14 g Protein: 4 g Sugars: 2 g Fiber: 0 g Sodium: 620 mg

481. Traditional English Mac N' Cheese

Servings: 12   Cooking Time: 1 Hour 20 Minutes
Ingredients:
- 2 lb. elbow macaroni
- ¾ C. butter
- ½ C. flour
- 1 tsp. dry mustard
- 1½ C. milk
- 2 lb. Velveeta cheese, cut into ½-inch cubes
- Salt and freshly ground black pepper, to taste
- 1½ C. cheddar cheese, shredded
- 2 C. plain dry breadcrumbs
- Paprika, to taste

Directions:
Set the temperature of   Grill to 350 degrees F and preheat with closed lid for 15 minutes.   In a large pan of lightly salted boiling water, cook the macaroni for about 7-8 minutes.   Drain the macaroni well and transfer into a large bowl.   Meanwhile, in a medium pan, melt 8 tbsp. of butter over medium heat.   Slowly, add flour and mustard, beating continuously until smooth.   Cook for about 2 minutes, beating continuously.   Slowly, add milk, beating continuously until smooth.   Reduce the heat to medium-low and slowly, stir in Velveeta cheese until melted.   Stir in salt and black pepper and remove from heat.   Place cheese sauce over cooked macaroni and gently, stir to combine. Place the macaroni mixture into greased casserole dish evenly and sprinkle with cheddar cheese.   In a small frying pan, melt remaining 4 tbsp. of butter.   Stir in

breadcrumbs and remove from heat.   Place breadcrumbs mixture over cheddar cheese evenly and sprinkle with paprika lightly.   Arrange the casserole dish onto the grill and cook for about 45-60 minutes, rotating the pan once halfway through.   Serve hot.

Nutrition Info: Calories per serving: 914; Carbohydrates: 99.9g; Protein: 37.2g; Fat: 42.3g; Sugar: 12g; Sodium: 1600mg; Fiber: 4.1g

482. Braised Pork Carnitas

Servings: 6   Cooking Time: 3 Hours
Ingredients:
- 3 lb. pork shoulder, sliced into cubes
- 2 tablespoons pulled pork dry rub
- 1 cup chicken broth
- 2 tablespoons olive oil
- Corn tortillas
- 3 jalapeno pepper, minced
- Cilantro, chopped
- Fresh cheese, crumbled
- Red onion, sliced

Directions:
Turn on your wood pellet grill.   Set it to 300 degrees F. Sprinkle the pork cubes with the dry rub.   Place in a Dutch oven.   Pour in the chicken broth.   Add the Dutch oven on top of the grill.   Open the sear slide. Bring to a boil.   Cover the Dutch oven and seal the sear slide.   Simmer for 2 hours and 30 minutes. Uncover and open the sear slide.   Bring to a boil. Take the Dutch oven off the grill. Set aside.   Pour the olive oil into a pan over medium heat.   Fry the pork for 10 minutes.   Top the corn tortillas with the pork cubes and the rest of the ingredients.

Nutrition Info: Calories: 250 Fat: 13 g Cholesterol: 40 mg Carbohydrates: 18 g Fiber: 2 g Sugars: 4 g Protein: 13 g

483. Bourbon Whiskey Sauce

Servings: 3   Cooking Time: 45 Minutes
Ingredients:
- cups ketchup
- 1/4 cup Worcestershire sauce
- 3/4 cup bourbon whiskey
- 1/3 cup apple cider vinegar
- 1/2 onions, minced
- 1/4 cup of tomato paste
- cloves of garlic, minced
- 1/2 tsp Black pepper
- 1/2 cup brown sugar
- 1/2 Tbsp Salt
- Hot pepper sauce to taste
- Tbsp Liquid smoke flavoring

Directions:

Preheat your grill for indirect cooking at 150°F   Place a saucepan over grates, then add the whiskey, garlic, and onions.   Simmer until the onion is translucent. Then add the other ingredients and adjust the temperature to Smoke. Simmer for 20 minutes. For a smooth sauce, sieve.
Nutrition Info: Per Serving: Calories: 107kcal, Carbs:16.6g Fat: 1.8g, Protein:0.8g

484. Smoked Hot Paprika Pork Tenderloin

Servings: 6   Cooking Time: 2 ½ To 3 Hours
Ingredients:
- 2-pound pork tenderloin
- 3/4 cup chicken stock
- 1/2 cup tomato-basil sauce
- 2 tbsp smoked hot paprika (or to taste)
- 1 tbsp oregano
- Salt and pepper to taste

Directions:
In a bowl, combine the chicken stock, tomato-basil sauce, paprika, oregano, salt, and pepper together.   Brush over tenderloin.   Smoke grill for 4-5 minutes. Pre head, lid closed for 10-14 minutes   Place pork for 2 ½ to 3 hours.   Rest for 10 minutes.
Nutrition Info: Calories: 360.71 Cal Fat: 14.32 g Carbohydrates: 3.21 g   Protein: 52.09 g Fiber: 1.45 g

485. Fennel And Almonds Sauce

Servings: 4   Cooking Time: 10 Minutes
Ingredients:
- 1 cup fennel bulb
- 1 cup olive oil
- 1 cup almonds
- 1 cup fennel fronds

Directions:
In a blender place all ingredients and blend until smooth Pour sauce in a bowl and serve

486. Smoked Chuck Roast

Servings: 6   Cooking Time: 5 Hours
Ingredients:
- 3 lb. chuck roast
- 3 tablespoons sweet and spicy rub
- 3 cups beef stock, divided
- 1 yellow onion, sliced

Directions:
Add the chuck roast to a baking pan.   Coat with the sweet, spicy rub.   Cover with foil. Refrigerate and marinate overnight.   Set the wood pellet grill to smoke. Preheat it to 225 degrees F.   Add the chuck roast to the grill.   Close the lid.   Smoke the chuck roast for 3 hours.   Brush with 1 cup beef stock every 1 hour.

Add the onion slices to a baking pan.   Pour the remaining beef stock.   Transfer the chuck roast on top of the onions.   Increase the heat to 250 degrees F.   Smoke for 3 hours.   Cover the chuck roast with the foil.   Smoke for another 2 hours and 30 minutes.   Let the chuck roast rest for 10 minutes.   Serving Suggestion: Serve with mashed potatoes.
Nutrition Info: Calories: 201 Fat: 13 g Cholesterol: 71 mg Carbohydrates: 0 g Fiber: 0 g Sugars: 0 g Protein: 21 g

487. Keto Quiche

Servings: 6   Cooking Time: 45 Minutes
Ingredients:
- 12 tbsp unsalted butter (soften)
- 12 large eggs
- 8 ounces grated cheddar cheese (divided)
- 4 ounces cream cheese
- ½ tsp salt or to taste
- ½ tsp ground black pepper or to taste
- 1 yellow onion (diced)
- 1 green bell pepper (chopped)
- 3 cups broccoli florets (chopped)
- 1 tbsp olive oil

Directions:
Preheat the grill to 325°F with the lid closed for 15 minutes.   Heat up the olive oil in a skillet over high heat.   Add the chopped onion, broccoli, and green pepper. Cook for about 8 minutes, stirring constantly. Remove the skillet from heat.   Process the egg and cheese in a food processor, adding the melted butter in a bit while processing.   Combine 4ounce grated cheddar cheese, salt, and pepper in a quiche pan.   Toss the cooked vegetable into the pan and mix.   Pour the egg mixture over the ingredients in the quiche pan. Sprinkle the remaining grated cheese over it.   Place the pan in the preheated grill and bake for 45 minutes. Remove and transfer the quiche to a rack to cool.   Slice and serve.
Nutrition Info: Calories: 615 Total Fat: 54.7 g Saturated Fat: 30.1 g Cholesterol: 494 mg Sodium: 804 mg Total Carbohydrate 8.1 g Dietary Fiber 1.9 g Total Sugars: 3.6 g Protein: 25.4 g

488. Crispy Fish Sticks

Servings: 6   Cooking Time: 5 Minutes
Ingredients:
- Olive oil
- 1 ½ lb. halibut, sliced into strips
- 1/2 cup all-purpose flour
- Salt and pepper to taste
- 2 eggs, beaten
- 1 1/2 cup panko breadcrumbs

- 2 tablespoon dried parsley
- 1 teaspoon dried dill weed

Directions:
Preheat the wood pellet grill to high for 15 minutes while the lid is closed. Pour olive oil to a pan. Add pan on top of the grill. Add flour, salt and pepper to a bowl. Mix well. Add the eggs to another bowl. In another bowl, mix the breadcrumbs and herbs. Dip the fish strips in the flour mixture, eggs and breadcrumb mixture. Place in oil and fry for 5 minutes or until golden. Tips: Beat the egg white first until frothy before stirring in egg yolk. This makes it easier for breadcrumbs to stick to the fish.

489. Smoked Tomato Cream Sauce

Servings: 1   Cooking Time: 1 Hour 20 Minutes
Ingredients:
- 1 lb beefsteak tomatoes, fresh and quartered
- 1-1/2 tbsp olive oil
- Black pepper, freshly ground
- Salt, kosher
- 1/2 cup yellow onions, chopped
- 1 tbsp tomato paste
- 2 tbsp minced garlic
- Pinch cayenne
- 1/2 cup chicken stock
- 1/2 cup heavy cream

Directions:
Prepare your smoker using directions from the manufacturer. Toss tomatoes and 1 tbsp oil in a bowl, mixing, then season with pepper and salt. Smoke the tomatoes placed on a smoker rack for about 30 minutes. Remove and set aside reserving tomato juices. Heat 1/2 tbsp oil in a saucepan over high-medium heat. Add onion and cook for about 3-4 minutes. Add tomato paste and garlic then cook for an additional 1 minute. Add smoked tomatoes, cayenne, tomato juices, pepper, and salt then cook for about 3-4 minutes. Stir often. Add chicken stock and boil for about 25-30 minutes under a gentle simmer. Stir often. Place the mixture in a blender and puree until smooth. Now squeeze the mixture through a sieve, fine-mesh, to discard solids and release the juices, Transfer the sauce in a saucepan, small, and add the cream. Simmer for close to 6 minutes over low-medium heat until thickened slightly. Season with pepper and salt. Serve warm with risotto cakes.
Nutrition Info: Calories 50, Total fat 5g, Saturated fat 1g, Total carbs 2g, Net carbs 2g, Protein 0g, Sugar 0g, Fiber 0g, Sodium: 69mg

490. Smoking Burgers

Servings: 8   Cooking Time: 40 Minutes
Ingredients:

- For the topping:
- 3 apples, peeled and cut into slices
- 75g blueberries
- 25g salted butter
- 2 tablespoons maple syrup
- For the cake:
- 75g butter, cut into cubes
- 75g organic virgin coconut oil, cut into cubes
- 100g cane sugar
- 2 large free-range eggs, beaten
- 75g buckwheat flour
- 75g ground almonds
- 1/2 teaspoon bicarbonate of soda
- 1 teaspoon baking powder
- 1 teaspoon cinnamon

Directions:
Preheat oven to 180°C. Caramelize the apples. Add the blueberries last. Set aside. Place the sugar, butter and coconut oil into a mixing bowl and cream until pale and fluffy. Gradually add the beaten eggs, adding a bit of flour if the mixture begins to curdle. Continue to beat the mixture until fluffy. Fold in the remaining flour, ground almonds, baking powder and cinnamon. Transfer the apple and blueberry mixture into the bottom of a greased Bundt cake mold, leveling well with the back of a spoon. Then pour the cake mixture over the top. Bake for about 40 minutes or until a skewer comes out clean. Leave to cool. Delicious served with Greek yogurt.
Nutrition Info: Calories: 275 Cal Fat: 10 g Carbohydrates: 31 g   Protein: 14 g Fiber: 4 g

491. Beets And Greens With Lemon-dill Vinaigrette

Servings: 4   Cooking Time: 1 Hour
Ingredients:
- 1½ pounds small beets, with fresh-looking greens still attached if possible
- ½ cup plus 2 tablespoons good-quality olive oil
- Salt and pepper
- 3 tablespoons fresh lemon juice
- 2 tablespoons minced fresh dill

Directions:
Start the coals or heat a gas grill for medium to medium-low direct cooking. Make sure the grates are clean. Cut the greens off the beets. Throw away any wilted or discolored leaves; rinse the remainder thoroughly to remove any grit and drain. Trim the root ends of the beets and scrub well under running water. Pat the leaves and beets dry. Toss the beets with 2 tablespoons of the oil and a sprinkle of salt until evenly coated. Put the beets on the grill directly over the fire. (No need to wash the bowl.) Close the lid and cook, turning them every 5 to 10 minutes, until a knife inserted in the center goes through with no resistance, 30 to 40 minutes total. Transfer to a plate and let sit until cool enough to handle. Toss the beet greens in the reserved bowl to coat in oil. Put the

greens on the grill directly over the fire. Close the lid and cook, tossing once or twice, until they're bright green and browned in spots, 2 to 5 minutes total. Keep a close eye on them; if they're on too long, they'll crisp up to the point where they'll shatter. Transfer to a plate.   Put the remaining ½ cup oil and the lemon juice in a serving bowl and whisk until thickened. Stir in the dill and some salt and pepper. Peel the skin from the beets and cut into halves or quarters. Cut the stems from the leaves in 1-inch lengths; cut the leaves across into ribbons. Put the beets, leaves, and stems in the bowl and toss with the vinaigrette until coated. Serve warm or at room temperature. Or makeup to several hours ahead, cover, and refrigerate to serve chilled.

Nutrition Info: Calories: 73 Fats: 3.8 g Cholesterol: 0 mg Carbohydrates: 9.6 g Fiber: 3.6 g Sugars: 2 g Proteins: 2.2 g

492. Dinner Rolls

Servings: 12   Cooking Time: 10 Minutes
Ingredients:
- 2 tablespoon active dry yeast
- 1/3 cup vegetable oil
- 1 1/10 cup warm water (115 degrees F)
- 1/4 cup sugar
- 1 egg, beaten
- Pinch salt
- 3 1/2 cups all-purpose flour
- Cooking spray

Directions:
Set the   wood pellet grill to 400 degrees F.   Preheat for 15 minutes while the lid is closed.   Use a stand mixer to mix dry yeast, oil, warm water, and sugar.   Let it rest for 10 minutes.   Stir in the egg, salt, and flour.   Spray cast iron pan with oil.   Knead the dough and shape into 12 balls.   Place the balls on the pan.   Let rest for 10 minutes.   Bake in the wood pellet grill for 10 minutes.

Nutrition Info: Calories: 77 Fats: 1.6 g Cholesterol: 1 mg Carbohydrates: 13 g Fiber: 0.5 g Sugar: 1.4 g Protein: 2.7 g

493. Wood Pellet Grill Chicken Flatbread

Servings: 6   Cooking Time: 30 Minutes
Ingredients:
- 6 mini breads
- 1-1/2 cups divided buffalo sauce
- 4 cups cooked and cubed chicken breasts
- For drizzling: mozzarella cheese

Directions:
Preheat your pellet grill to 375 - 400F.   Place the breads on a surface, flat, then evenly spread 1/2 cup buffalo sauce on all breads.   Toss together chicken breasts and 1 cup buffalo sauce then top over all the breads evenly.   Top each with mozzarella cheese. Place the breads directly on the grill but over indirect heat. Close the lid.   Cook for about 5-7 minutes until slightly toasty edges, cheese is melted and fully hated chicken.   Remove and drizzle with ranch or blue cheese.   Enjoy!

Nutrition Info: Calories 346, Total fat 7.6g, Saturated fat 2g, Total Carbs 33.9g, Net Carbs 32.3g, Protein 32.5g, Sugars 0.8g, Fiber 1.6g, Sodium 642mg, Potassium 299mg

494. Satisfying Veggie Casserole

Servings: 10   Cooking Time: 3 Hours
Ingredients:
- 5 tbsp. olive oil, divided
- 6 C. onions, sliced thinly
- 1 tbsp. fresh thyme, chopped and divided
- Salt and freshly ground black pepper, to taste
- 1 tbsp. unsalted butter
- 1¼ lb. Yukon gold potatoes, peeled and 1/8-inch thick slices
- ½ C. heavy cream
- 2¼ lb. tomatoes, cut into ¼-inch thick slices
- ¼ cup black olives, pitted and sliced

Directions:
In a large cast iron pan, heat 3 tbsp. of oil and over high heat and cook onions, 1 tsp. of thyme, salt and black pepper for about 5 minutes, stirring occasionally.   Add the butter and cook over medium heat for about 15 minutes.   Reduce the heat to low and cook for about 10 minutes.   Set the temperature of   Grill to 350 degrees F and preheat with closed lid for 15 minutes. Meanwhile, in a bowl, add potatoes slices, cream, 1 tsp. of thyme, salt and black pepper and toss to coat.   In another bowl, add tomato slices, salt and black pepper and toss to coat.   Transfer half of the caramelized onions into a small bowl.   In the bottom of the cast iron pan, spread the remaining onion slices evenly and top with 1 layer of potatoes and tomatoes.   Drizzle with 2 tbsp. of cream from potato mixture and 1 tbsp. of olive oil.   Sprinkle with a little salt, black pepper and ½ tsp. of thyme.   Spread remaining caramelized onions on top, followed by potatoes, tomatoes and olives. Drizzle with remaining cream from the potatoes and remaining tbsp. of olive oil.   Sprinkle with a little salt, black pepper and remaining ½ tsp. of thyme.   With a piece of foil, cover the cast iron pan tightly.   Place the pan onto the grill and cook for about 2 hours.   Remove from grill and uncover the cast iron pan.   Now, set the temperature of   Grill to 450 degrees F.   Place the cast iron pan, uncovered onto the grill and cook for about 25-30 minutes.   Remove from grill and serve hot.

Nutrition Info: Calories per serving: 158; Carbohydrates: 14.8g; Protein: 2.3g; Fat: 11.1g; Sugar: 5.8g; Sodium: 65mg; Fiber: 3.2g

495. North American Pot Pie

Servings: 10   Cooking Time: 1 Hour 25 Minutes
Ingredients:
- 2 tbsp. cornstarch
- 2 tbsp. water
- 3 C. chicken broth
- 1 C. milk
- 3 tbsp. butter
- 1 tbsp. fresh rosemary, chopped
- 1 tbsp. fresh thyme, chopped
- Salt and freshly ground black pepper, to taste
- 2¾ C. frozen chopped broccoli, thawed
- 3 C. frozen peas, thawed
- 3 C. chopped frozen carrots, thawed
- 1 frozen puff pastry sheet

Directions:
Set the temperature of Grill to 375 degrees F and preheat with closed lid for 15 minutes. In a small bowl, dissolve cornstarch in water. Set aside. In a pan, add broth, milk, butter and herbs over medium heat and bring to a boil. Add the cornstarch mixture and stir to combine well. Stir in salt and black pepper and remove from the heat. In a large bowl, add the vegetables and milk sauce and mix well. Transfer mixture into a cast iron skillet. With the puff pastry, cover the mixture and cut excess from edges. Place the skillet onto the grill and cook for about 80 minutes. Remove the pan from grill and set aside for about 15 minutes before serving. Cut the pie into desired-sized portions and serve.
Nutrition Info: Calories per serving: 257; Carbohydrates: 26.1g; Protein: 7.6g; Fat: 14g; Sugar: 5.8g; Sodium: 408mg; Fiber: 4.7g

496. Sweet Potato Spiced Fries

Servings: 4   Cooking Time: 30 Minutes
Ingredients:
- 1 tsp of kosher salt
- 2 Tbsp of olive oil
- 1 tsp of paprika
- 1/2 tsp of cumin, ground
- 2 pounds of sliced sweet potatoes
- 1 tsp of brown sugar, light
- 1 tsp of chili powder
- 1 tsp of garlic powder

Directions:
Mix the brown sugar, paprika, garlic powder, chili powder, salt, and cumin in a bowl. Mix the sliced potatoes and oil in a separate bowl, then add the brown sugar mixture and toss well. Pour the coated potatoes into a roasting pan and roast until it is brown and tender. This will take about 15-20 minutes. Serve as soon as possible.
Nutrition Info: Per Serving: Calories: 177.85kcal, Protein: 23.9g, Carbs: 21.9g, Fat: 39.8g.

497. Summer Treat Corn

Servings: 6   Cooking Time: 20 Minutes
Ingredients:
- 6 fresh whole corn on the cob
- ½ C. butter
- Salt, to taste

Directions:
Set the temperature of Grill to 400 degrees F and preheat with closed lid for 15 minutes. Husk the corn and remove all the silk. Brush each corn with melted butter and sprinkle with salt. Place the corn onto the grill and cook for about 20 minutes, rotating after every 5 minutes and brushing with butter once halfway through. Serve warm.
Nutrition Info: Calories per serving: 334; Carbohydrates: 43.5g; Protein: 7.7g; Fat: 18.1g; Sugar: 7.5g; Sodium: 171mg; Fiber: 6.3g

498. Berry Smoothie

Servings: 1   Cooking Time: 1 Minutes
Ingredients:
- 2 scoops Protein Powder
- 2 cups Almond Milk
- 4 cups Mixed Berry
- 2 cups Yoghurt

Directions:
First, place mixed berry, protein powder, yogurt, and almond milk in the blender pitcher. Then, select the 'smoothie' button. Finally, pour the smoothie to the serving glass.
Nutrition Info: Calories: 112 Fat: 2 g Total Carbs: 26 g Fiber: 0 g Sugar: 0 g Protein: 1 g Cholesterol: 0

499. Smoked Garlic White Sauce

Servings: 2   Cooking Time: 1 Hour
Ingredients:
- 2 cups hickory wood chips, soaked in water for 30 minutes
- 3 whole garlic heads
- 1/2 cup mayonnaise
- 1/3 cup sour cream
- 1 juiced lemon
- 2 tbsp apple cider vinegar
- Salt to taste

Directions:
Cut garlic heads to expose the inside and place in a container, microwave-safe, with 2 tbsp water. Microwave for about 5-6 minutes on medium. Preheat your grill. Place garlic heads on a shallow foil "boat" and place it on the grill. Close the grill and cook for about 20-25 minutes until soft completely. Remove and cool. Transfer into a blender then add the

remaining ingredients. Process until smooth.   Serve immediately or store in a refrigerator for up to 5 days.
Nutrition Info: Calories 20, Total fat 0g, Saturated fat 0g, Total carbs 8g, Net carbs 8g, Protein 0g, Sugar 0g, Fiber 0g, Sodium: 45mg

500. Beer-braised Pork Shank

Servings: 6   Cooking Time: 23 Minutes
Ingredients:
- 2 Tbsp Flour
- Kosher salt
- Ground black pepper
- 2 Tbsp olive oil
- 2 Tbsp butter
- 1 medium onion, diced
- 2 carrots, trimmed and diced
- 1 Tbsp garlic, minced
- 1 cup dried mushrooms
- 2 cup beef broth
- 2 Tsp chili powder
- 2 thyme sprigs
- 2 Tsp coffee, instant
- 1 Tbsp Worcestershire sauce
- 12 oz dark beer, porter
- 2 dried bay leaves

Directions:
Preheat wood pellet smoker-grill to 300ºF with the cover of the grill closed for 10 minutes.   Hold pork shank together with a butcher string and sprinkle pepper and salt over it.   Place a Dutch oven on the cooking grid. Add oil and pork shanks. Cook shank until brown on both sides.   Remove shanks from heat and transfer to a plate.   Sauté onions, carrots, and garlic in Dutch oven until tender, about 8 minutes.   Mix in beef broth, beer, and Worcestershire sauce to the sautéed vegetables. Increase the temperature and bring to boil. Allow simmering at Medium temperature until one-third of the liquid is gone.   Add tomato paste, coffee, thyme, chili powder, and bay leaves.   Transfer pork shanks from the plate into the Dutch oven and scoop sauce atop it. Cook shanks until tender, about 3 hours.   Combine in a bowl, butter, and flour. Add the flour mixture in the last hour to thicken the sauce.   Take out bay leaves and thyme springs. Cut out butcher's string. Serve pork shank with gravy atop it and garnish with parsley.
Nutrition Info: Per Serving: Calories: 85kcal, Carbs: 2.0g, Fat: 3.5g, Protein: 7.0g

CPSIA information can be obtained
at www.ICGtesting.com
Printed in the USA
LVHW010513260121
677404LV00009B/625